Reader's Digest Guide to Skin Care

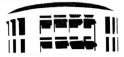

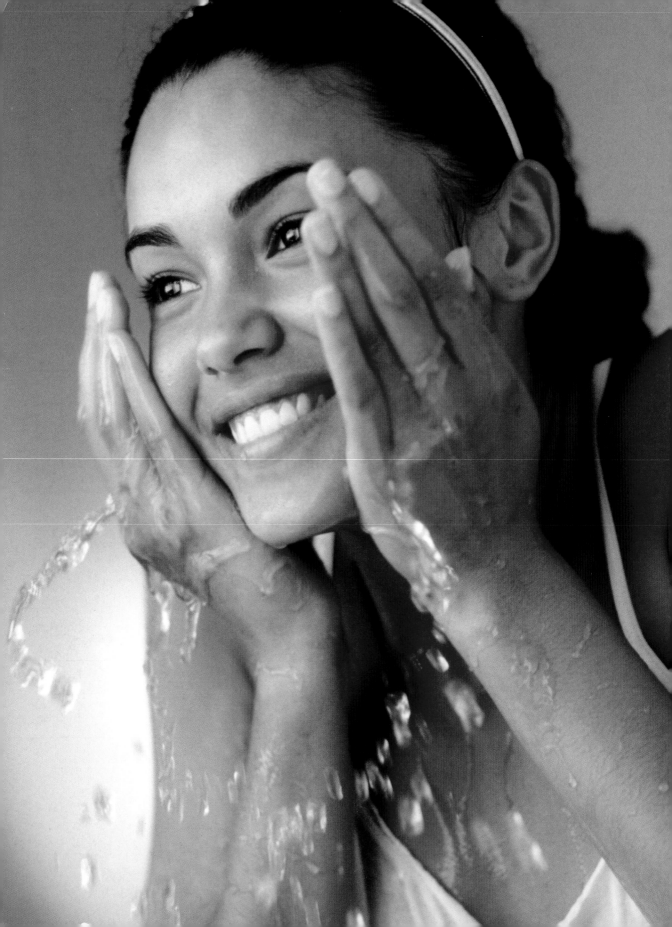

Reader's Digest Guide to
Skin Care

Professional Secrets and Natural Treatments for Glowing, Youthful Skin

SUSAN C. TAYLOR, M.D.,
AND VICTORIA HOLLOWAY BARBOSA, M.D., M.P.H., M.B.A.

Foreword by William D. James, M.D.
Paul Gross Professor of Dermatology, The University of Pennsylvania

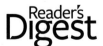

Reader's
Digest

The Reader's Digest Association, Inc.
Pleasantville, New York/Montreal/London/Singapore/Mumbai

A READER'S DIGEST BOOK

Copyright © 2009 Quantum Publishing Ltd
This edition published by The Reader's Digest
   Association, Inc., by arrangement with
   Quantum Publishing Ltd

FOR QUANTUM PUBLISHING
Project Editor Samantha Warrington
Designer Andrew Easton
Production Rohana Yusof
Publisher Anastasia Cavouras

FOR READER'S DIGEST
U.S. Project Editor Siobhan Sullivan
Canadian Project Editor Jesse Corbeil
Canadian Project Manager Pamela Johnson
Project Designer Jennifer Tokarski
Senior Art Director George McKeon
Executive Editor, Trade Publishing Dolores York
Associate Publisher Rosanne McManus
President and Publisher, Trade Publishing
   Harold Clarke

Library of Congress Cataloging in Publication Data:
Taylor, Susan C.
   Reader's Digest guide to skin care : Professional
Secrets and Natural Treatments for Glowing, Youthful
Skin / Susan C. Taylor and Victoria Holloway Barbosa.
      p. cm.
 ISBN 978-1-60652-129-8 (hardcover)
 ISBN 978-1-60652-105-2 (paperback)
1. Skin--Care and hygiene--Popular works. I.
Barbosa, Victoria Holloway, 1968- II. Reader's Digest
Association. III. Title. IV. Title: Guide to skin care.
 RL87.T385 2009
 616.5--dc22
                        2009030546

We are committed to both the quality of our products
and the service we provide to our customers. We value
your comments, so please feel free to contact us:

   The Reader's Digest Association, Inc.
   Adult Trade Publishing
   Reader's Digest Road
   Pleasantville, NY 10570-7000

For more Reader's Digest products and information,
visit our website:

www.rd.com (in the United States)
www.readersdigest.ca (in Canada)
www.readersdigest.co.uk (in the UK)
www.rdasia.com (in Asia)

Printed in Singapore

1 3 5 7 9 10 8 6 4 2 (hardcover)
1 3 5 7 9 10 8 6 4 2 (paperback)

NOTE TO OUR READERS
The information in this book should not be substituted
for, or used to alter, medical therapy without your
doctor's advice. For a specific health problem, consult
your physician for guidance.

To my wonderful family: my husband, Kemel Dawkins; my daughters, Morgan Elizabeth and Madison Lauren; my parents, Ethel and Charles Taylor; and my sister, Flora Taylor. To my extraordinary colleague and partner on this project, Dr. Victoria Holloway Barbosa, without whom the *Reader's Digest Guide to Skin Care* would not have been written.

– Susan C. Taylor

To my beloved family: my husband, Valdir; my daughter, Gabrielle Sophia; and my mother, Dorothy Holloway—with gratitude for your unwavering support, encouragement, and understanding. To my dear friend and esteemed colleague, Dr. Susan C. Taylor, who continues to be a tremendous inspiration.

– Victoria Holloway Barbosa

Contents

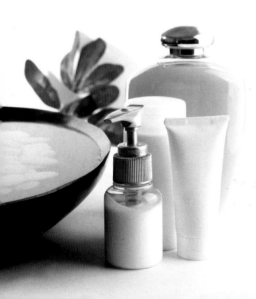

Foreword

Nearly everyone has encountered a problem with their skin that is medically important, unsightly, or just a nuisance. Melanoma and other skin cancers are occurring earlier in life and are rising in incidence yearly. Acne affects 85 percent of teenagers and now lasts more commonly into adult life. The environment is filled with a variety of hazards to skin health, including the always present and skin-damaging sun, as well as insects, germs, and poison ivy. As the population continues to age, there are more of us with skin that sags, wrinkles, and develops a large variety of spots. What are these new growths? Are they barnacles reflective of a long life or the next scary threat to your existence?

Dr. Susan C. Taylor and Dr. Victoria Holloway Barbosa provide a wonderful resource for you and your family to learn about your skin and its challenges. With colorful images, a straightforward style, and tips that will help you when preparing to see your doctor, this book is an invaluable resource. It also debunks common misconceptions, explaining for instance that the red nose of rosacea is not due to being an alcoholic and you can in fact remove that unsightly hair protruding from your mole without need for concern. Over-the-counter solutions are suggested to allow you to start to care appropriately for your skin problems while deciding whether or not to visit your doctor. The numerous options available today for cosmetic improvement can be bewildering. What are the details of how these various options work, when might they fit your needs, and what are the potential problems? This book will help you to get those answers and many more!

I am happy that this exciting and powerful resource is available to everyone. With the knowledge available from the trusted editors at Reader's Digest, combined with the book's engaging style and presentation, I believe that everyone can benefit from reading it. By understanding your body's largest organ more completely, you can better prevent problems, know when to seek medical advice, and become more well versed in possible treatment strategies.

William D. James, M.D.
Paul Gross Professor of Dermatology
The University of Pennsylvania

Introduction

We love skin. Each of us has dedicated our professional life to learning about it, caring for it, healing it, and teaching others about it. Skin care and disease management is really more than just our job as dermatologists. It is truly a lifelong passion, one that has united us not only as colleagues but also as long-time friends. *Reader's Digest Guide to Skin Care* is a manifestation of our delight in caring for others, our desire to empower people through education, and a profound respect for each other and our profession. We hope that our passion is evident to you as you read this book.

As dermatologists, we have treated thousands and thousands of people with skin disease. Some people we have cured. Others we have helped to manage diseases for which there is not yet a cure. Through these encounters we have heard countless questions that people have about their skin. And many of these questions get asked over and over again by different people. We know that if our patients have these questions, then other people do, too. With this book, we have tried to answer all of the common questions that we get asked every day, in order to answer them for you as well.

Every day we answer questions from our patients about the skin and how best to care for it. In this book we answer the most commonly asked questions for you, our readers.

We have created a book that stands apart from all the other skin care books on the shelf. This is because we have been able to combine our many years of expertise as board-certified dermatologists with our extensive experience in the cosmetics industry. With Dr. Taylor as the founder and CEO of a cosmetic product company and Dr. Barbosa as a former cosmetics industry executive for many years and now an industry consultant, we are in a unique position to provide a well-rounded view of the skin, useful products, pesky problems, and real solutions. This book is an indispensable reference. If you have questions about how your skin works, how to care for it, what might be wrong with it, how to treat it, or where to turn if you need professional help, we provide the answers here. We want to arm you with information and help you ask the right questions at the cosmetics counter and in the doctor's office.

How you use this book is up to you. You may want to read it cover-to-cover. *Reader's Digest Guide to Skin Care* provides a thorough overview of the skin, how best to care for it, common skin diseases, procedures, and information about how your overall health affects your skin. In essence, it provides you with a firm foundation of general knowledge. Alternatively, you may pick and choose which sections to read, selecting only those chapters or sections that are of interest to you at any point in time. Each section stands on its own and was written with this type of use in mind as well. We hope that you will refer to this book frequently as your different skin care needs arise.

Reader's Digest Guide to Skin Care is engaging, easy to read, and loaded with useful information that will give you the answers you need to better understand and care for your skin and your health.

Susan C. Taylor, M.D.
Victoria Holloway Barbosa, M.D., M.P.H., M.B.A.

1

How the Skin Works

Essential to your health, beauty, and well-being, your skin is an important part of who you are. There are many myths and much misinformation about your skin and its care. *Reader's Digest Guide to Skin Care* sets the record straight, starting with the basics. This chapter explains the functions and structure of the skin, and helps you understand the different types of skin specialists.

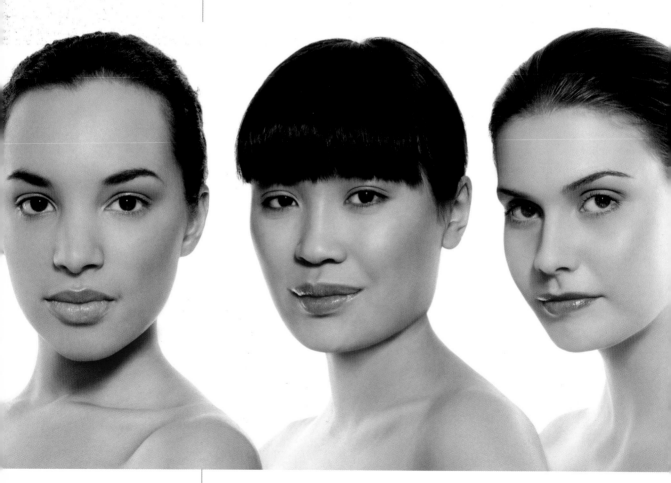

The physiological functions of the skin

You may often take your skin for granted and not realize all of the vital functions it performs. No one would deny that the heart is an organ essential to keeping us alive. Just like the heart, the skin is an organ crucial to your body's survival. The most important role that the skin plays is to protect you from the harsh and dangerous environment: everything from heat, humidity, and cold to chemicals, ultraviolet radiation, and microorganisms.

Your skin is a barrier

The skin is a waterproof barrier that seals the body from losses of fluid that could lead to dehydration and death. It resists invasion by various types of microorganisms such as bacteria, fungi, and viruses that cause infections and serious illness. The skin also blocks many chemicals and allergens from entering the body. It filters out the burning rays of the sun and protects our cells from cancer-causing radiation. It acts as a shock-absorber, cushioning internal organs from damage.

Keeping the skin healthy is very important given its wide range of critical activities. There are many ways that you can keep your skin's barrier function intact. Take the time to apply moisturizer when your skin is dry. Avoid things that disrupt the skin like harsh scrubs and vigorous scratching. And seek treatment for skin diseases promptly. With these steps, the skin will better protect you from the outside world.

Your skin is a thermostat

Whether you are lying on the beach in Rio de Janeiro or playing ice hockey in Anchorage, your body temperature remains constant. That is largely because your skin acts to cool the body down when it gets too hot and helps to warm the body when it gets too cold in order to maintain a temperature of approximately 98.6°F (37.0°C). So, your skin works like your home's

Skin Myth

True or False?
The skin is the body's largest organ.

True
The skin is both the largest and the heaviest organ. The liver is the second largest and heaviest organ.

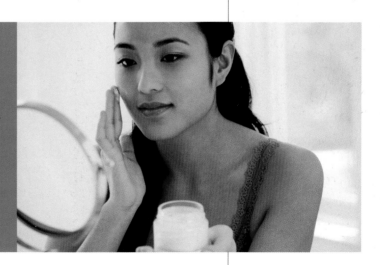

MOISTURIZE

Moisturizers help the epidermis stay soft and smooth by increasing or maintaining its water content.

They also help to maintain the skin's barrier function by preventing the cracks that are so common in dry, flaky skin.

For best results, apply moisturizer immediately after cleansing, while the skin is still damp.

thermostat does when it keeps the temperature inside constant despite fluctuations in the weather outside.

Your internal organs naturally generate heat as they function, including your muscles, your heart, and even your brain. When the outside temperature is higher than your body temperature and you are at risk for overheating, your skin produces sweat that evaporates from its surface and cools you down. Sweat is mostly water, so when you sweat a lot it is easy to become dehydrated. That is why it is important to drink water during and after exercise. Sweat also contains small amounts of waste products such as urea, lactic acid, and salts so its secondary role is elimination of waste from the body.

Your skin also helps to eliminate heat from the body through the dilation of the blood vessels. This allows more blood to flow to the surface of the skin where heat is given off. When the outside temperature is cold, these same vessels contract keeping more blood away from the surface of the skin to prevent heat loss. There are also tiny muscles in the skin that make your hairs stand up, which provides a layer of insulation against the cold.

> Sweating is normal when it is hot outside, when you are anxious, and during menopause. Unexplained sweating can be a sign of a problem with the thyroid or the nervous system.

Touch is one of the key ways a baby bonds with its parents, and it is even important for the baby's brain development.

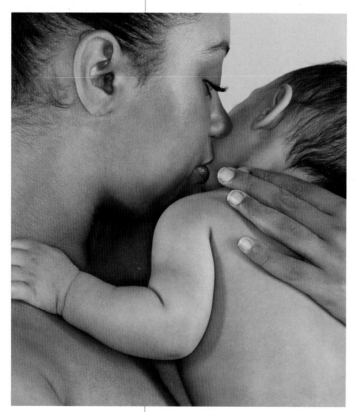

Your skin is a sensor

How do you know that your coffee is too hot to drink? Or that there is an ant crawling on your leg? Or that you have stepped on a thumbtack? Throughout your body, your skin has millions of receptors, or nerve endings that provide your sense of touch. Most people know that touch is one of the five senses, but did you know that there are different kinds of receptors to perceive different types of stimuli such as temperature, light touch, vibration, and pain?

These nerve endings in your skin transmit information along your nerves to your spinal cord and up to your brain, all within a fraction of a second. In this way you receive important information like the pleasure of another person's touch or the danger of a scalding hot frying pan or the cold air that requires you to put on a coat, and you can respond accordingly. Sometimes you respond to these sensations deliberately, after thinking about them. Other times you respond reflexively, without having to think first. This is a protective mechanism that allows you to respond to danger very quickly.

Some areas of the body have more sensory receptors than others. For instance, the finger tips have a lot of nerve endings and are able to perceive subtle touch but the lower back has relatively few and is not as sensitive. The lips, tongue, face, feet, and the genitals are other areas that also have a lot of nerve endings. Along with sight, smell, hearing, and taste, touch allows you to better understand, enjoy, and respond to your environment.

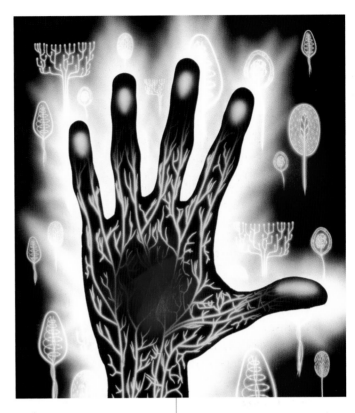

A network of receptors transmits impulses from the hand, along the nerves of arm, to the spinal cord, and then to the brain.

Your skin is a factory

Vitamin D helps you to form healthy bones, fortifies your immune system to fight cancers, and helps your body to prevent a variety of diseases such as depression and multiple sclerosis.

Did you know that your skin is your body's vitamin D production factory? Ultraviolet light penetrates the uppermost layer of the skin, the epidermis, where it stimulates the synthesis of this important vitamin. It is estimated that you need somewhere between five and thirty minutes of exposure to the sun twice per week to your face, arms, legs, or back to derive adequate sunlight to meet your vitamin D needs. People with brown skin produce less vitamin D than people with fair skin who are in the sun for the same amount of time. This is because the melanin that gives the skin its color also acts to filter the sun's light so vitamin D production takes longer.

If you do not spend time in the sun or if you are adequately protecting your skin from the sun in order to prevent skin cancer then you will need to obtain more of your vitamin D from your diet.

SKIN SOLUTION
People of color often need to take vitamin D supplements during seasons of temperate and cool weather to compensate for lower vitamin D production. Your doctor can check for vitamin D deficiency with a simple blood test.

The psychological functions of the skin
In addition to its physiological functions, our skin is an indicator of who we are. It is often a reflection of our identity and our individuality. We can

enhance our appearance through adornments such as makeup, tattoos, and piercings. How we style our hair and nails, which are formed from our skin, are two additional ways in which we express our identity. You might convey your outgoing, confident self with red nail polish one week and show your conservative or demure side the next week with a French manicure. You might display your creativity with blue hair dye in one phase of life, and cover your gray hair with brown hair color in another phase.

The skin is a window

How you feel on the inside can affect how your skin looks and functions on the outside. When you are happy and healthy, your skin tends to look its best. However, when you are under stress, or feeling anxious or depressed, skin diseases can flare, nails can become brittle, and hair can fall out in large amounts. The changes caused by your emotional state can actually alter the ability of the skin to function properly. For example, if you have a condition like eczema and it flares due to stress, your skin will be inflamed and the barrier function will be compromised.

As you can see, emotional well-being and our skin are closely related. They are also related through our sense of touch. It is the nerve fibers in the skin that allow us to perceive touch. Touch gives us the unique ability to connect with others on an emotional level and to share deeply with others. Deprivation of touch can lead to developmental, social, and psychological problems in children that can be long-lasting. As well as expressing comfort and caring, touch is inextricably entwined with pleasure and intimacy.

SKIN SOLUTION

Manage your daily stress effectively to help keep your skin looking its best. Balance work with time for family, friends, and fun. Eat a well-balanced diet and make time for exercise and sleep. Try meditation or listen to soothing music to help you relax.

LAYERS OF THE EPIDERMIS

Layer	Function
Stratum basale	The cells of this layer divide indefinitely to form daughter cells that rise through the epidermis. Basal cell skin cancers arise from this level.
Stratum spinosum	Synthesis of keratin proteins begins in this layer.
Stratum granulosum	Keratin and lipids that waterproof the skin are produced in this layer.
Stratum lucidum	This layer is mainly found on thick skin like the palms and soles and contains dead keratinocytes.
Stratum corneum	Contains 15 to 20 layers of dead skin cells that ultimately slough off.

The structure of the skin

There are two main layers of skin: the epidermis and the dermis. The third layer is the subcutaneous fat that is found underneath the dermis.

Epidermis

As the skin's outermost layer, the epidermis is the body's barrier against the outside world. This is a very important job for a part of the body that ranges in thickness from only 0.05 to 1.5 millimeters! To put this in perspective, a piece of paper is approximately 0.08 millimeters thick. There are four different types of cells in the epidermis.

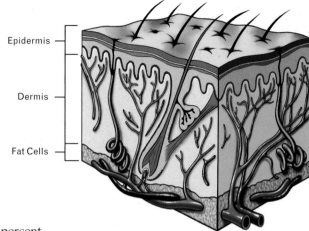

Epidermis

Dermis

Fat Cells

Keratinocytes are the most prevalent cells in the epidermis. These cells make up over 90 percent of the epidermal cells and are arranged in five layers that sit on top of the basement membrane, which separates the epidermis from the dermis below. These cells make keratins, the proteins that give strength to hair, skin, and nails. It takes approximately thirty days for new skin cells to form and move upward from the bottom to the top layer of the epidermis. You can think of keratinocytes as bricks that form the "wall" of the skin.

Melanocytes are cells that are found in the basal layer of the epidermis. The job of the melanocyte is to make melanin, the pigment that gives skin its color. Melanin is also found in the hair and in the irises of the eyes. There are actually two types of melanin. Eumelanin imparts brown and black color to the hair, skin, and eyes. Pheomelanin is red and is found on the lips and the genitals. It is also more abundant in the hair of redheads and the skin of people with red undertones. Melanin is the substance that provides the skin with protection from the sun.

Langerhan's cells are the third type of cell that populates the epidermis. These are cells that are part of the body's immune system. When a microorganism enters the skin, it is the Langerhan's cell that acts as the first line of defense by activating the rest of the body's immune system to fight off the invader.

Merkel cells are the fourth type of cell found in the epidermis. They are mainly found in its basal layer. The function of these cells is to act as receptors for light touch. In the epidermis, the keratinocytes, melanocytes, Langerhan's cells, and Merkel cells all work together to keep the skin healthy.

The layers of the skin work together to provide a healthy covering for your body. Similar to a double layer cake, the skin is made of two major layers, the upper layer is called the epidermis and the lower layer is the dermis. Beneath the dermis is a layer of fat.

Skin Myth

True or False?
People with fair skin have fewer melanocytes than people with darker-colored skin.

False
Everyone has the same number of melanocytes, regardless of skin color.

Dermis

The dermis provides the support structure of the skin. It consists of two layers, the papillary dermis, which is closest to the epidermis, and the reticular dermis below. The dermis is comprised of collagen, elastin, and extracellular matrix (ECM), which acts as the glue that holds everything together. There are fibroblast cells which produce the collagen, elastin and ECM, and also immune cells that protect the skin by moving into and out of the dermis. Hair follicles, sweat glands, nerves, and blood vessels are also found in the dermis.

> While your dermis is not visible, it is important to the overall appearance of your skin because it provides the strength and elasticity that keep your skin looking firm and youthful.

Fibroblasts are the cells that are responsible for producing the collagen and elastin that provide support, strength, and elasticity to the skin. They also make the ECM in which everything is contained. When the skin is injured or cut, fibroblasts begin to produce collagen to repair it. If too much collagen is produced, hypertropic scars, or keloidal scars result. On the other hand, as we age and expose our skin to ultraviolet sunlight, collagen is lost and elastin fibers are broken down. Fibroblasts also produce less new collagen and elastin. This results in fine lines, wrinkles, sagging, and thin, fragile skin.

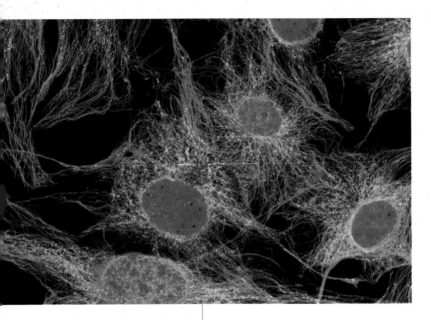

A confocal light micrograph of fibroblast cells.

Hair follicles are structures that originate in the dermis and extend through the epidermis to the skin's surface. You can think of them as small tubes in the dermis. At the bottom of the tube is the hair root that actually makes a hair. When a hair is made, it grows up and out of the hair follicle. The opening of the follicle is commonly referred to as a pore. While most people want to minimize the appearance of these openings, they actually don't change size.

Sebaceous, apocrine, and eccrine glands are located within the dermis. Sebaceous and apocrine glands are located adjacent to hair follicles and empty into them. The oil from the sebaceous gland and the apocrine sweat travel up the follicle and are deposited on the surface of the skin. The oil acts as the skin's natural moisturizer. Bacteria attracted to the apocrine sweat produce body odor, and these glands are primarily located under the arms and in the genital area. The eccrine sweat gland duct passes through the dermis and opens directly onto the skin's surface where it deposits sweat. Eccrine sweat glands are key in helping the body regulate temperature. They are located all over the body and are especially numerous on the palms of the hands and soles of the feet.

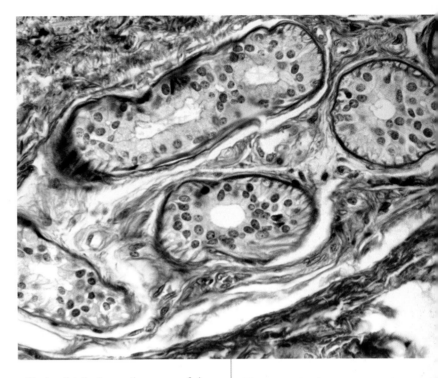

Nerves in the dermal layer of the skin allow us to sense pain, temperature, and itch. Others allow us to detect pressure and vibration. If you think about the areas of the body that are most sensitive, they are the areas that have the greatest number of nerves: the fingers, hands, feet, face, and genitals.

The sweat gland is composed of a secretory portion (upper left) and several excretory ducts (bottom left to top right).

Blood vessels provide oxygen and nourishment to the skin cells. These vessels are also important in temperature control with cooling of the body occurring when the blood vessels enlarge to allow enhanced flow of blood to the skin. In contrast, when exposed to cold, blood vessels constrict or close, decreasing blood flow and conserving heat to help keep you warm.

Subcutaneous layer

The subcutaneous fat lies below the dermis. It is also called adipose tissue. This layer helps to insulate the body against heat gain and loss. This fat layer also serves as an energy reserve; its lipids can be burned by the body to form energy.

SKIN SOLUTION

Many people complain that their nails are too brittle. Biotin is one of the B vitamins, and it can help this condition. Look for supplements that contain 2500 micrograms of Biotin, and take one daily.

The structure of nails

Nails provide protection for the fingers and toes and increase the sensation of touch. Fingernails and toenails grow very slowly: it requires 3 to 6 months for a fingernail to be completely replaced and 12 to 18 months for the complete replacement of a toenail. Nails grow faster in the summer than they do in other seasons.

When you think about your nail, you probably think about the hard clear surface that you can polish and trim. This is actually called the nail plate and is made of keratin. There are several other structures that together make up the nail unit. The nail bed is the soft pink skin under the nail plate. The lunula is the white half-moon that you can see at the base of the nail plate. The nail folds are areas where skin overlaps the nail plate. The area along the sides of the nail from which a "hang nail" can form are called the lateral nail folds, and the protective cuticle area is called the proximal nail fold. The eponychium is the dead skin in the cuticle area that some peole trim during a manicure or pedicure, and the paronychium is the living skin in the cuticle area. The hyponychium is the area under the nail where dirt collects; you may clean it with an orange stick. The matrix is the "root" of the nail from which the nail plate grows. It sits deep within the proximal nail fold.

The nail plate is curved, which allows it to be securely embedded into the proximal and lateral nail folds, providing strong attachments and sealing the nail from the environment. The curvature of the toenail is greater than that of the fingernail, which accounts for the occurrence of more "hang nails" in this area. Just as in the skin, melanocytes are present in the nail matrix. In people with darker skin tones, nail matrix melanocytes contain mature packages of melanin, called melanosomes. They sometimes cause pigmented streaks within the nail. The nail matrix of Caucasians is not pigmented and lacks mature melanosomes.

Brittle nails are a common complaint. Nails contain a great deal of water, but when they become dehydrated and their percentage of water drops below 7 percent, the nail becomes brittle and breaks. In contrast to this, when the water content of nails rises above 30 percent, they become opaque and soft.

Avoid trimming cuticles during a manicure in order to reduce the risk of infection. Push them back instead.

The nail plate is formed by several compact layers of keratin that give it strength.

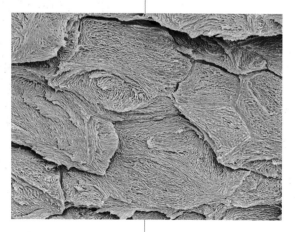

The structure of hair

When you consider your hair, you probably think about the hair on your head or maybe those annoying ones that grow on your chin. In fact, there are approximately 5 million hair follicles all over the body, with only 80,000 to 150,000 follicles on your scalp. Hair is made at the bottom of the hair follicles in an area called the hair root or bulb. The matrix cells in this region actively divide and produce the cortical cells which become the substance of the hair fiber itself. Along the length of the hair shaft there are three layers: the central hair shaft fiber, the middle inner root sheath, and the outer root sheath. The central hair shaft is continuous with the inner root sheath within the follicle. The hair shaft itself is composed of three layers: the protective outer cuticle, the cortex, and sometimes an inner medulla. The hair follicle is important for many reasons, and its shape contributes to the structure of the hair. A curved follicle contributes to the tight curl of African hair; straight Asian hair follicles give rise to straight Asian hair.

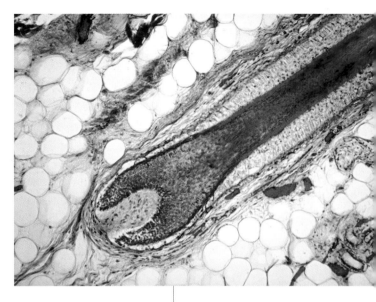

The bulb lies at the base of the follicle. It is the region in which hair is formed.

The phases of hair growth

Once formed, hair undergoes three phases of growth: the anagen, catagen, and telogen phases. During the anagen phase, active growth occurs for 2 to 8 years. This phase is followed by the brief catagen rest phase, for a few weeks, after which the 2 to 4 month shedding called the telogen phase occurs. A telltale sign of a telogen hair is a white ball on the end of the hair. At any point in the hair-growth cycle, 85 to 90 percent of the 150,000 scalp hairs are growing; the others are resting or shedding.

Many people complain that their hair just does not grow. In fact, hair length corresponds to the amount of time the hair spends in the anagen growth phase and the rate of growth African hair tends to grow more slowly, and Asian hair tends to grow the most rapidly. Caucasian hair tends to fall somewhere between the two. Also hair breakage occurs more readily in some individuals than in others. For example, African hair is more prone to breakage than Caucasian hair owing to its tightly coiled shape.

Why light skin and dark skin react differently

Have you ever wondered why your Irish skin develops blistering sunburn while your best friend's Indian skin tans when you both sit on the beach for 30 minutes? Or have you pondered why your Australian-born grandmother has had three basal cell carcinomas but your southern Italian grandfather has never had skin cancer? It is all related to the amount of melanin that you have in your skin. Melanin acts as a great sunscreen, protecting the skin from burning UV rays, from skin cancer, and from premature aging. People with darker skin tones have larger melanosomes; these are full of melanin, which absorbs more ultraviolet light than the smaller melanosomes in fair-skinned individuals of northern European descent.

Skin Myth

True or False?
Some people have hair that stays the same length and doesn't grow.

False
Different people's hair grows at different speeds and for different lengths of time. Also some people's hair breaks off more easily than others.

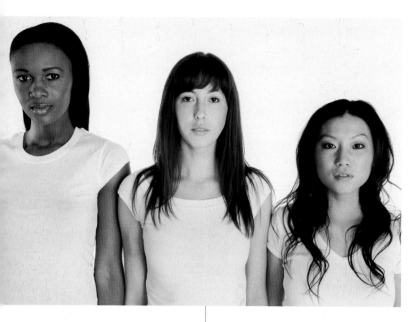

Studies have demonstrated that very darkly pigmented skin has a natural sun protection factor (SPF) of 13, as compared to the natural SPF of 3 in fair, white skin. In a study of Asian skin, Japanese women with more melanin, as evidenced by their darker complexions, reacted less severely to the sunlight.

However, this does not mean that darker skin tones, when exposed to sunlight for a long time, will not burn. In general melanin also serves to provide protection from premature aging and from skin cancers.

Different skin tones react differently to sunlight due to the varying amounts of melanin.

Normal variation in skin pigmentation

Have you noticed that the skin on your face is not the same color as the skin on your arms, or that the skin in the genital region is a different color than the skin on your hands? It is normal for people to have variation in their skin's pigmentation, with some areas appearing lighter or darker than others on different parts of the body. This is especially true for people with skin of color.

Eyelid pigmentation

Do you have dark circles under your eyes that just won't go away? There are many causes for the appearance of dark circles, but one of the most common causes is genetic. Have a look at your mother and father. If they have the same dark circles, then you have your answer.

Periorbital hypermelanosis is a common condition, also called periorbital hyperpigmentation. This condition can be seen in people of any ethnic background, but is more common in people with olive, tan, or brown skin.

SKIN SOLUTION

Get plenty of rest to help minimize the appearance of dark circles under the eyes. Cold compresses can help to reduce puffiness. Eye creams can help to improve the appearance of fine lines. Not much can be done to change the genetic component of dark under eye circles, so just thank your mom or dad!

Face and body skin pigmentation

Pigmentary demarcation lines (PDLs) are one of the most commonly occurring forms of pigmentation variation. These are areas that represent changes in the amount of melanin pigment in the skin with an abrupt transition from darker to lighter skin tone. Although they have been seen in Caucasians, they are much more common in people with skin of color; and one study has estimated that approximately 75 percent of African Americans have at least one PDL.

These lines can arise at any time from birth onward. They are often noted to arise during pregnancy. This is especially true of linea nigra which appears on the abdomen. Pregnant women may also notice darkening of the tissue around the nipple, the areola. It is believed that the elevated estrogen levels from the pregnancy may cause these two conditions. Until recently there were five types of PDL's described, named Types A through E.

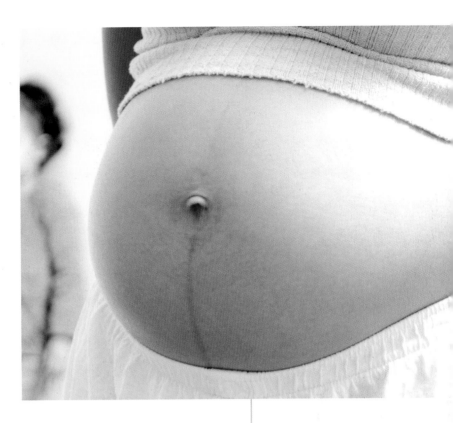

Linea nigra commonly occurs on a pregnant woman's abdomen, usually during the second trimester.

More recently, three additional patterns of hyperpigmentation have been been described on the face in an Indian population, which some consider Types F through H. PDLs are commonly referred to as Futcher's lines or Voight's lines. There is no way to prevent or to remove pigmentary demarcation lines.

PIGMENTARY DEMARCATION LINES	
Type	**Description**
A	Lines along the length of the arms and possibly extending to the chest
B	Lines along the back of the thighs and possibly extending to the ankles
C	Straight or curved line along the mid-chest
D	Straight line along the spine
E	Light spots from the clavicles to the nipples
F	"V" shaped hyperpigmentation extending from the outer eye to the temple
G	"W" shaped hyperpigmentation extending from the outer eye to the temple
H	Linear hyperpigmentation from the corners of the mouth down to the chin

Nail pigmentation

The pigmented nail streak is another common variant that is considered normal, especially in individuals with darker skin tones. Longitudinal melanonychia and pigmented nail band are other names for this condition, which is characterized by a tan or brown band that runs the length of the nail. Over 50 percent of African Americans above the age of 50 have at least one nail with this streak. The degree of nail pigmentation is increased in patients with darker skin pigmentation. It is important to note that pigmented nail bands are not common in Caucasian skin and may be a sign of a skin cancer. Any Caucasian with longitudinal melanonychia should be evaluated by a dermatologist.

Although you may not like them, dark lines or even light lines on various parts of the body may be entirely normal.

Hand and foot pigmentation

Dark spots on the palms of the hands and the soles of the feet are another normal pigmentary variant in dark-skinned people. They are called melanotic macules of the palm and soles. These lesions vary in size and shape but are always flat. They can usually be distinguished from moles by a trained eye. It is important to distinguish melanotic macules from nevi, particularly atypical appearing nevi. This is because acral melanomas that occur on the hands and feet are more common in people of African descent.

Oral pigmentation

Oral pigmentation can be seen on the gums, the roof of the mouth, the inside of the cheeks, or on the tongue of people of color. This finding is usually completely normal in this population, and is very common. For instance, oral pigmentation occurred in 93 percent of dark-skinned Brazilian children compared to 12 percent in fair-skinned Brazilian children in one study. The color of the oral pigmentation can vary from light brown to dark brown or can even appear blue-black, and does not require any treatment.

Is important to keep in mind that oral pigmentation is sometimes more than just an incidental finding. It can result from taking some medications, like minocycline, or from smoking cigarettes. It can also result from silver fillings, caps,

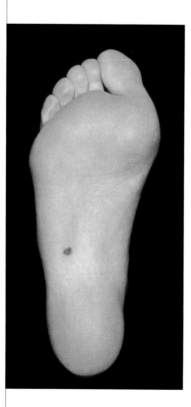

Brown spots on the soles may be moles or harmless melanotic macules. Any changing brown spots on the palms or soles should be evaluated immediately.

or crowns. Dentists call these spots amalgam tattoos. While uncommon, it is possible to get moles, and even skin cancers in the mouth. These lesions are usually raised. While oral pigmentation is usually nothing to worry about, it is important to bring it to your doctor's attention.

Who's who in skin care

Whether you have a question about your skin, you are looking for preventative skin care, or you are having a problem like a rash or a changing mole, it is important to know where to go for help. This section provides a guide to the different types of professionals who help to keep skin healthy and looking its best.

The dermatologist

A dermatologist is a medical doctor who specializes in the diagnosis and management of skin diseases. These professionals have had extensive education, including four years of college and four years of medical school. They then receive hands-on training, first for one year of internship in either internal medicine, surgery, pediatrics, or a combination of the three. They then complete three years of dermatology training in the United States, and four years in Canada. This training is called residency. Some dermatologists go on for additional fellowship training as well. Areas of sub-specialty training include pediatric dermatology, dermatopathology, Moh's surgery, laser surgery, and procedural dermatology.

In the United States, anyone who has completed a dermatology residency training program is then eligible to sit for the American Board of Dermatology examination, commonly referred to as "the boards." These people are called "board eligible." Once the doctor passes the examination he or she is then "board certified." Most countries have similar certifying examinations. In Canada dermatologists are certified by the Royal College of Physicians and Surgeons of Canada.

The primary care doctor

Primary care doctors include internists, family practitioners, general practitioners, and

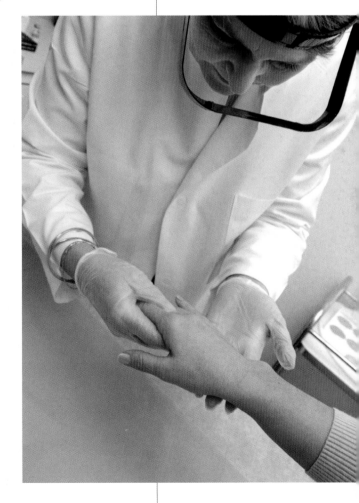

A dermatologist examining a woman's hand. She is wearing a visor that magnifies the skin.

pediatricians. For many people, their trusted primary care doctor is the first stop for all health related questions, including skin questions. Some primary care doctors perform full-body skin examinations, provide an opinion on whether a growth is benign or if it needs a biopsy, and will treat routine conditions like acne and eczema. The amount of skin care a primary care doctor provides depends on the level of her education and training in the skin and its diseases, her comfort in managing these conditions, and often on her patient load.

A primary care doctor who takes care of many sick patients may refer even basic skin conditions to the dermatologist to have more time to focus on her patients who are more sick. A great doctor knows when to treat the patient and when to refer them to a dermatologist for specialist care. As with your dermatologist, knowing that your primary care doctor is board-certified will provide you with a certain level of confidence about her amount of training and ongoing medical education.

Physician's assistants receive on-the-job specialty training from their supervising physicians.

The physician's assistant

Physician's assistants, or PAs, are commonly employed in dermatologists' offices. They are health care providers who have had two to three years of formal health education after college, including both classroom work and clinical rotations in several medical specialties. Unlike physicians, PAs do not complete a residency after completing their education. They are trained by the physician who employs them in the specialty of that physician. They may work in different specialties during different parts of their career. It is, of course, in a doctor's best interest to train his PA well since the doctor is still ultimately responsible for the care the PA provides and for the health of the patient. While PAs have been an integral part of the health care system in the United States for many years, other countries, including Canada, are also starting to have similar training programs.

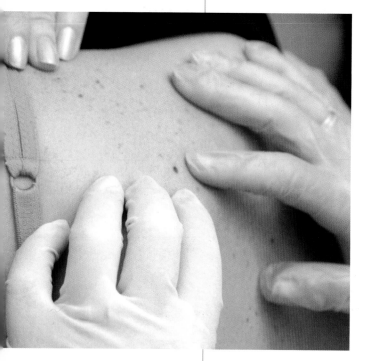

Physician's assistants work with doctors to provide medical treatments and perform procedures.

The nurse practitioner

Nurse practitioners (NPs) are found in many countries throughout the world, and are sometimes also called advanced practice nurses. They are registered nurses who obtain masters or doctoral level education in nursing and pass a certifying examination. Unlike PAs, NPs may obtain board certification in a specific field of medicine, although dermatology is not currently one of these fields. In some places NPs are able to practice completely independently, in others they must have an association with a physician. NPs are able to diagnose and treat medical conditions and often manage routine skin diseases. They take your medical history, perform physical examinations, diagnose and treat medical conditions, and prescribe medications. NPs most commonly work in primary care fields but may occasionally be found in the dermatologist's office as well.

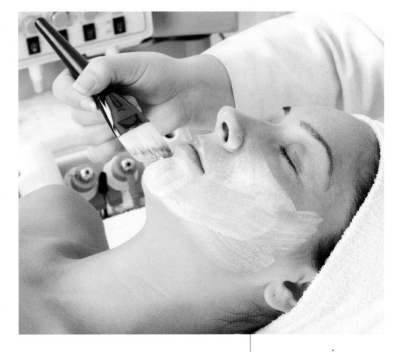

Estheticians provide facials, which are a good way to cleanse the skin, exfoliate dead cells, and remove comedones, also known as blackheads and whiteheads.

The esthetician

Estheticians are people who are trained in providing skin care services and recommending skin care products. In addition to obtaining their classroom education at beauty school, these professionals are required to complete hundreds of hours of training and have to pass an examination.

Estheticians often work in physicians' offices and are also found in salons and spas. They provide services, such as facials, superficial chemical peels, microdermabrasion, waxing, body wraps, etc. While estheticians do not diagnose or treat medical problems, they are often the first ones to point out something questionable on your skin and may refer you to a dermatologist for evaluation.

The beauty advisor

Beauty advisors are found in cosmetics retail stores and at the cosmetics counters in department stores. They are sales people who are trained in the uses and benefits of the skin care and cosmetics products that they represent. They may offer product advice, consultation sessions, and makeovers to guide you in choosing from the seemingly countless number of products at the cosmetics counter. A great beauty advisor is able to educate you and help you make good product choices. She helps you find what you need and is not just making a sale.

It is very important to ask your skin doctor if he is board-eligible or board-certified in dermatology.

A dermatologist provides a full-body skin examination on a young patient.

Skin examinations

Regularly scheduled skin examinations are the key to the early detection of skin problems such as cancers and other diseases. Found early, skin cancers are usually easily managed. However, left unchecked, they can cause the destruction of large amounts of tissue, and this will require larger operations, resulting in more obvious scarring, and can even cause death.

Professional examinations

Professional examinations are performed routinely by dermatologists and also by some primary care doctors, PAs and NPs. You should plan to have a professional examination annually, unless your physician suggests that you need to be screened more frequently. This may happen if you have a lot of moles that look atypical to the naked eye or under the microscope, if you have a history of skin cancer, or a strong family history of skin cancer.

A full-body skin examination is just that, so prepare yourself for the office visit. In order to perform this exam properly, the doctor needs to be able to see all of your skin, so you will be asked to change into a gown. Some doctors will have you leave your undergarments on at first, others will ask that you remove them before the exam begins. Either option is fine, it just depends on the style of the doctor and your comfort level as a patient.

In addition to looking at all of the obvious parts of your body your doctor may look in areas you don't expect. For instance, your doctor will look

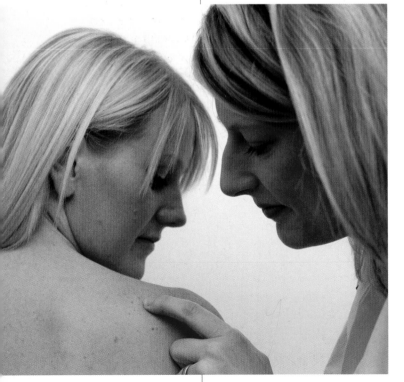

through your hair to evaluate your scalp. You may want to skip using hairspray on the day of the examination, and wear your hair in a style that allows for easy visibility of the scalp. If you wear a wig, try not to be embarrassed if the doctor asks you to remove it.

The full-body skin examination will also include a look in your mouth, so it would be best if you get rid of your chewing gum before the office visit starts. Your doctor will want to have a look at the skin in the groin and around the rectum. Some doctors will defer this exam if a woman has had a recent genital examination by an obstetrician/gynecologist, or primary care doctor.

Also, your doctor will want to be able to see your fingernails and toenails easily, so remove your nail polish prior to your visit.

The doctor's toolbox

During an evaluation by a dermatologist, there are several different kinds of tests that might be performed on the skin to aid in diagnosis of your condition. Some of the most common ones are discussed here.

Dermoscopy

Dermoscopy is used by some dermatologists to help diagnose skin conditions, to distinguish benign growths from malignant ones, and to help monitor changes in lesions. Oil is placed on the skin to aid in the visualization provided by the handheld microscope.

Skin scrapings

Superficial layers of the epidermis are removed by gently scraping the surface of the skin with a scalpel blade. This procedure is usually painless. The dead skin,

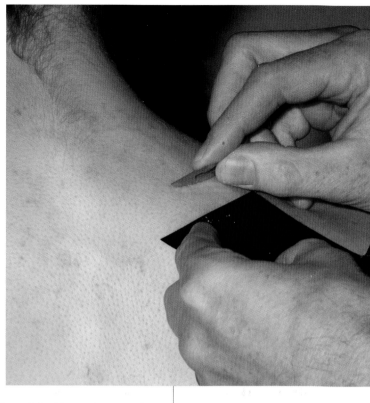

called scales, that are collected are placed on a glass slide. Depending on the organism that is suspected, the scales will be treated with a chemical and then visualized under the microscope.

Several infectious conditions can be diagnosed with this test. If the physician sees evidence of mites burrowing beneath the stratum corneum, he or she might scrape a little harder and this procedure might be a little uncomfortable. If he or she sees blisters that are suggestive of an infection with a herpes virus such as herpes simplex or varicella, he or she may nick the blister, unroof it, and scrape the underlying skin. This too, can be a little uncomfortable.

Organisms detected by skin scrapings include:
- Fungi
- Scabies mites
- Demodex mites
- Herpes viruses

Your dermatologist may make a diagnosis using her naked eye and her sense of touch, however, additional testing is sometimes required.

The benefits usually outweight the risks of a skin biopsy, which include bleeding, infection, and scarring.

Wood's lamp examinations

Wood's lamp examinations are used to evaluate pigmentation problems and to help diagnose some infections. The lights in the examination room will be turned out and your doctor will examine you with a black light.

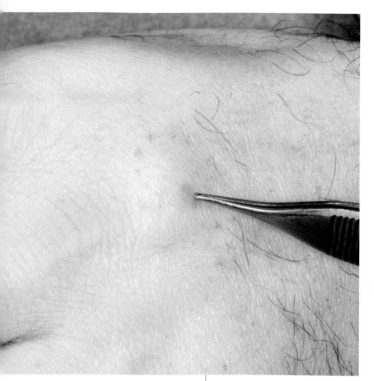

Skin biopsies

When more information is needed about the skin than can be discerned with the naked eye, your doctor may suggest a skin biopsy. This entails taking a small piece of skin to look at under the microscope. The good news is that the worst part of the biopsy is the preparation. Numbing medicine is usually given as an injection into the area of interest. In addition to a small needle stick, you will feel burning for a few seconds as the numbing medicine goes into the skin. It works right away, so you will not feel pain during the biopsy. Some people do feel slight pressure, but this is not uncomfortable. There are different types of skin biopsies. The physician will determine which one is best for your condition.

Monthly self-exams combined with annual professional exams will help you identify cancers and other problems early.

Shave biopsy utilizes a scalpel or razor blade to plane off a small area of the skin. No stitches are needed with this type of biopsy. Sometimes a doctor wants to make sure that he or she removed the entire lesion in question. In this instance, the scalpel or razor blade is used to take a deeper, more extensive amount of skin. This is sometimes called a saucerization, a shave excision, or a deep shave.

Punch biopsy requires a tool that looks like a miniature apple corer. It is a small, round razor blade that comes in diameters ranging from 2 to 12 mm. Usually doctors use the 2, 3, or 4 mm punches. This tool allows the doctor to obtain a cylindrical core of skin, and usually one stitch is placed, although larger punches require more stitches.

SKIN SOLUTION

Self-examinations are an important way to detect changes in your skin at an early stage, when problems like skin cancer are easier to treat. If you examine your skin on the same day of each month it will be easier to remember.

Excisional biopsy is performed when a doctor wants to be sure that an entire lesion is removed at the time of the biopsy. A scapel is used to cut out skin around the area of interest, usually in the shape of an ellipse, and stitches are used to bring the skin back together.

What happens when the numbing medicine wears off? This is a common question. Usually the numbing medicine loses its effect after about an hour or two. Most people only have slight discomfort at the biopsy site and don't require any pain reliever. If you do experience pain you should take acetaminophen. Aspirin and ibuprofen containing pain relievers can thin the blood and increase your risk of bleeding from the biopsy site.

Self-examinations

Self-examinations are also important and should be carried out more frequently than the professional examination. Each person should perform a self-examination monthly. Eventually this will become a habit but you may need to remind yourself at first. If you examine yourself on the same day of each month it will be easier to remember.

For instance, the first day of every month can be your self-exam day. Set this as a recurring appointment on your calendar. It also makes sense to pair your skin exam with your monthly breast exam so that you remember to do both.

Self exams are easier to do if you have a partner. The other person will help remind and motivate you. He or she will also be able to double-check the hard-to-see areas that might be tricky to do on your own. This is a very personal examination, so choose your partner wisely. If you don't have someone to partner up with it's no problem. You can absolutely see everything you need to by yourself.

Skin cancers can occur in people of all skin tones and ethnic backgrounds. Everyone should perform a monthly self-examination.

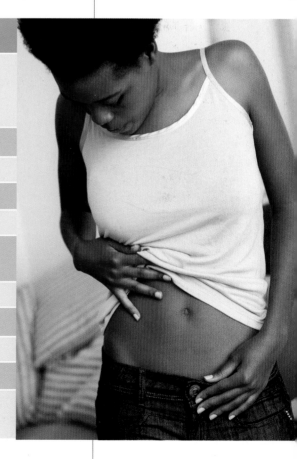

RISK FACTORS FOR SKIN CANCER

Several risk factors increase your chance of developing skin cancer. If you meet any of these criteria, you should be particularly diligent about your skin exams. You are at higher risk for skin cancer if you have:

- A personal history of skin cancer

- A family history of skin cancer

- Fair skin

- Sun-sensitive skin that burns easily

- Significant recent or past exposure to ultraviolet (UV) rays from the sun, tanning beds, or sun lamps

- Ever experienced severe, or numerous sunburns

- Atypical or unusual looking moles

- 50 or more moles

- History of X-ray treatments

- An immune system that is weakened by medication or disease

How to perform a self-examination

1. Work your way through your scalp by parting your hair in sections and examine the scalp between the hairs. Use a large mirror like your bathroom mirror to see the front half of your scalp. Then, turn your back to the large mirror and position the handheld mirror in front of you so that you can see the back of your scalp in the big mirror.
2. Look at your face, ears, and the front of your neck in the large mirror.
3. Look in your mouth with a flashlight and the handheld mirror. Look at the roof of your mouth, the sides of the mouth, the top of your tongue and under the tongue.
4. Look at your chest, abdomen, arms, underarms, and hands, using the mirror to see areas that you can't see directly. Don't forget to lift the breasts to see the skin underneath.
5. Look at the fronts of your legs, bottom of your feet, and in between your toes.
6. Utilize one or both mirrors to check the back of your neck, upper and lower back, buttocks, and the backs of your legs.
7. Use the hand mirror to check the skin around your genitals and anus. You may need to use the flashlight for better visualization. While this may seem awkward, it is important to remember that skin cancers can appear anywhere on the body.

What to look for during a self-examination

The purpose of your self-examination is to identify skin conditions as early as possible. This is especially true for skin cancers and pre-cancers, but this is an opportunity to identify any skin problem you are having. You do not have to worry about actually figuring out if a spot is harmless or cancerous. Your goal is to be able to point out new spots, spots that have changed, or spots that leave you feeling uneasy to your doctor so that he or she can make a judgment about whether or not further work-up or treatment is necessary.

During your self-examination write down anything you see, including moles, growths, bumps, scabs, and spots that bleed or won't heal. For each spot you see, you want to pay attention to several factors like location, size, shape, color, and any irregularities. You can use a body mole map to document what you see by diagramming and listing your findings. A free body mole map is available for download from the American Academy of Dermatology website.

Point out moles that have changed to your doctor so that she can examine them and determine if they need to be biopsied.

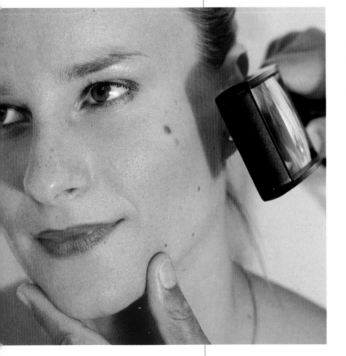

Use a new sheet for each exam, date it and save the charts together. This way it will be easy for you to compare findings from month to month. If you do have new or changing lesions, you should not wait for your next annual professional examination to bring them to your doctor's attention. You should make an appointment to see your dermatologist right away so that he or she can evaluate the areas.

Melanoma screening

There are several different types of skin cancers, and a detailed discussion follows in chapter 5. It is important to know that one of the key diseases that you are looking for during your self-examination is melanoma. It tends to be much more aggressive than other common skin cancers, with a greater likelihood of spreading to other parts of the body and higher mortality rates. When found at the earliest stage these cancers have a 99 percent 5-year survival rate. Unfortunately when they are found later and have spread to distant organs, the 5-year survival rate drops to 18 percent. Detecting melanoma early is critical to a patient's chances of survival.

While melanoma is uncommon in children, its incidence is on the rise. Keep an eye out for unusual growths on your children as well as yourself.

Several organizations, including the American Academy of Dermatology and the Skin Cancer Foundation, educate people about the "ABCDE's" of melanoma. These are the characteristics that you should look for when you look at a mole to specifically to determine if it is suspicious for melanoma. If you have any spots that have any of the features listed, be sure to point those out to your physician. Just because you have a mole that has one or more of these features does not mean you have melanoma; it just means that you need to be evaluated by a professional.

ABCDE's OF MELANOMA SCREENING		
Letter	**Characteristic**	**Meaning**
A	Asymmetry	One half of the lesion does not look like the other half
B	Border	The edge of the growth is not smooth but may be jagged, notched or scalloped
C	Color	Pigmentation is not consistent throughout the mole and may have different shades of tan, brown, black, white, red or blue
D	Diameter	The mole is more than 6 mm at its widest point
E	Evolving	Changes in size, shape, or color of existing moles

2

Beauty & Skin Care

Taking good care of your skin is important for your health and for your sense of well-being. When you look good, you feel good. There is an endless array of skin care products to choose from, each claiming to make us look better, healthier, and younger. How do you begin to sort through the choices? This chapter provides a comprehensive guide to thinking about your skin care.

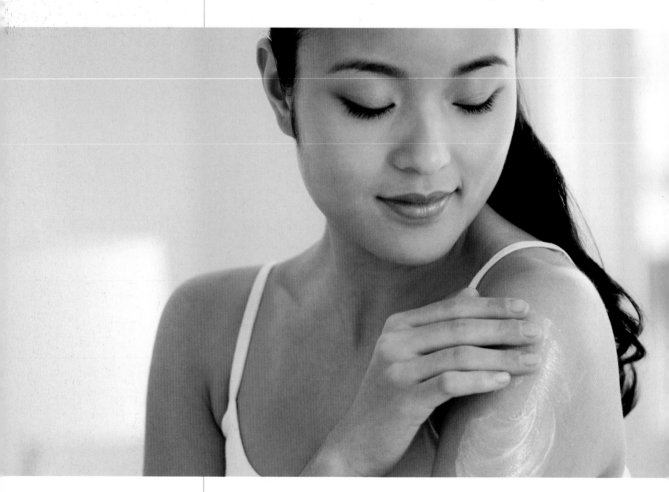

Your facial skin type

What is your facial skin type? This can be a confusing question because there is no single, universally accepted skin-typing system. Sometimes skin type refers to the amount of sebum production, that is whether the skin is dry or oily. Sometimes it refers to the amount of pigment in the skin or how it reacts to sunlight. Doctors, authors, and even cosmetics companies use the term "skin type" in different ways.

Despite the confusion, it is important for you to know your skin type in the broadest sense. You must understand your skin's unique needs in order to take care of it properly and to select the right skin care products.

Dry, oily, combination, and normal skin

Many skin products, particularly cleansers and moisturizers, are formulated for skin based on the amount of sebum it produces. Do you know if your skin is dry, oily, combination, or normal? If not, there is a simple test for finding out. Wash your face with a mild cleanser and wait one hour. If your skin feels tight or looks flaky, you have dry skin. If you are already a little shiny, you have oily skin. If your skin feels healthy and is neither flaky nor oily, it is normal. And if your skin is different in different areas, you have combination skin.

Sensitive skin

Sensitive skin reacts easily to skin care products. You may notice redness, itching, tingling, or burning after the application of different products. Sometimes the sensation is more than just reactivity: it is the result of irritation from a product or even an allergy to an ingredient.

Once you have determined that you have sensitive skin, be very careful in selecting the right skin care products. Use gentle, alcohol-free, and unperfumed products. Avoid using facial scrubs, and soaps that are drying as these can be too harsh for sensitive skin. Always perform a patch test whenever using a new kind of cosmetic to avoid an allergic reaction.

WHAT IS YOUR SKIN TYPE?

To fully identify your skin type, you must ask six questions:

- Is my skin dry, oily, both, or neither?
- Is my skin sensitive to certain products or environmental factors?
- Do I develop facial acne easily?
- Do I tend to develop dark spots easily?
- How sensitive am I to sunlight?
- Am I starting to show signs of aging?

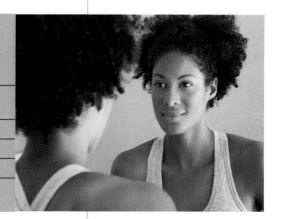

Acne-prone skin

Do you occasionally develop blackheads, whiteheads, pimples, or painful cysts? If so, you have acne. This is a skin disease that can be treated with over-the-counter and prescription medications. A discussion of acne and its treatments follows in the next chapter.

What is important to know here is that if your skin is acne-prone, you need to look for skin care products that do not make your acne worse. Some over-the-counter skin care products contain ingredients that help to treat acne. You should use moisturizers and make up products that say "non-comedogenic."

Sun-sensitive skin

All skin types benefit from sun protection. It reduces the risk of skin cancer, delays photoaging, and helps to minimize pigmentation problems. How much sun protection you need depends on how your skin responds to sunlight. If you never burn, you may be able to wear a moisturizer with

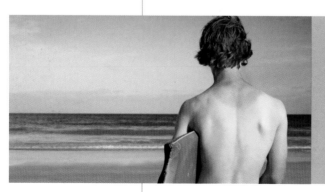

SUN-SENSITIVE SKIN

The Fitzpatrick Skin Type Classification system labels skin types from 1 (always burns) to 6 (never burns). This classification is often misused as a classification for skin color. Although the two are related, they are not the same. The Fitzpatrick scale is used mostly by dermatologists as part of an evaluation of the skin.

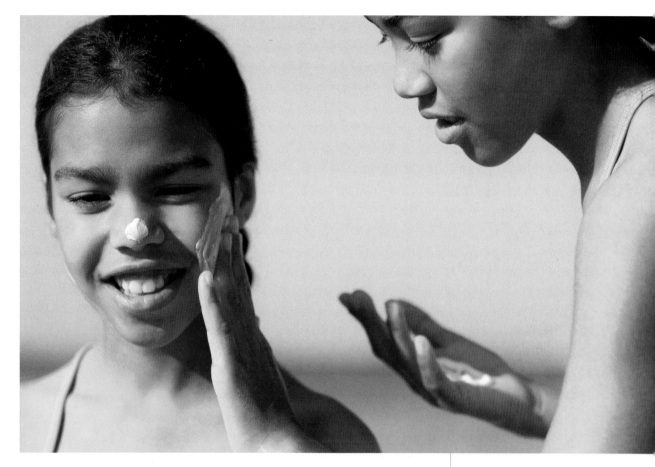

SPF 15 protection. If you burn easily, you may need an SPF of 30 or higher on a daily basis. How does your skin respond to the sun's rays on a summer day? Do you burn quickly? Do you tan, then burn with prolonged exposure? Are you someone who never burns?

Your answer depends largely on how much pigmentation your skin has. Fair-skinned people tend to burn easily, while richly pigmented brown skin takes longer to burn or may only burn seldomly.

Apply sunscreen 30 minutes before going into the sun, then reapply it every two hours and every time you get out of the water.

Hyperpigmentation-prone skin

It is important to determine the underlying cause of your hyperpigmentation in order to prevent it. For instance, if you get dark spots from acne, then it is important to treat the acne so that you don't continue to get new spots as you treat the old ones. A detailed discussion of hyperpigmentation follows later in this chapter.

HYPERPIGMENTATION-PRONE SKIN

If the answer to any of these questions is yes, you have hyperpigmentation-prone skin.

- When you get a pimple, do you develop a dark spot that lasts for several weeks or months?
- Has your skin ever darkened after using a product that was irritating?
- Do you develop blotchy tan or brown pigmentation after exposure to the sun?

Aging skin

Everyone's skin ages. We may not be happy about it, but it is a reality. Two main factors contribute to how your skin ages. The first is genetics, which play a role in chronological aging. You can largely thank your parents for how well your skin holds up to the test of time. The second is the environmental exposures your skin has had. Sun exposure and tobacco use are the two environmental conditions that cause the most aging. You are solely responsible for this part of the aging process!

Over time, the skin starts to lose its firmness and elasticity. This is because the collagen and elastin found in the dermis decrease as we get older. This leads to wrinkles and sagging skin. Also, the skin produces less sebum, so it becomes drier. In addition, skin cells don't slough off as easily, giving a more ashen appearance. The epidermis becomes thinner, so the skin may take on a papery appearance, and underlying blood vessels become more apparent. A loss of the fat under the skin gives the face a more drawn-in, hollow appearance.

Your lifestyle choices play a big role in how your skin ages. Prolonged, repeated exposure to sunlight causes photoaging. Effects of this can include brown spots on the face, wrinkles, a yellowish tint to the skin, broken blood vessels, easier bruising, and the development of a leather-like texture to the skin. Tobacco use also accelerates aging. In short, chronic sun exposure and tobacco use make you look even older than you already are. Who needs that?

Your facial skin care needs may change over the seasons. For instance, you may have dry skin in the winter and normal skin in the summer. Or you may have normal skin in your 30s and 40s but then it may become more dry in your 50s. This means that you will need to reassess your skin type and your skin's needs both seasonally, and as you get older. Your skin-care-product use should change as your skin changes.

SKIN SOLUTION

Follow these tips to keep your skin looking its youthful best: wear sunscreen every day, avoid smoking, drink plenty of water, and eat foods rich in antioxidants, like berries, grapes, tomato, broccoli, and green tea.

Sun exposure ages the skin prematurely and can lead to skin cancer.

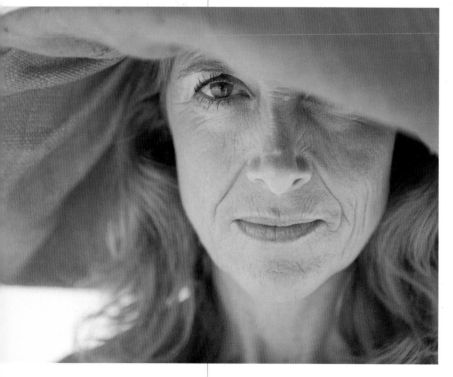

Products for your facial skin care

There are four steps to consider in caring for your face: cleansing, treating special problems, moisturizing, and protection. These steps should be repeated morning and night.

Step 1: Cleansing

Simplicity is the key here. You need to find a good cleanser that your skin responds well to, and stick with it. There are excellent cleansers available in all price ranges. Just because one is more expensive than another does not mean that it is better for your skin.

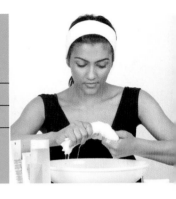

FOUR SIMPLE STEPS TO SKIN CARE

1. **Cleanse**
2. **Treat**
3. **Moisturize**
4. **Protect**

Skin cleansing should be done every day as it removes oils, dirt, makeup, and dead skin cells from the surface of the face. Water alone is not enough to rinse the unwanted debris from your face. When you pour vegetable oil and water in a glass, the oil just sits on top of the water. Similarly, if you just splash your face with water, the oils remain on the skin because the oil and water do not mix.

Skin cleansers are made of surfactants. Surfactants are substances that have two parts: a hydrophilic, or water-loving, end and a hydrophobic, or water-repelling, end. The water-resistant end of the detergent molecules is attracted to the oils on the skin and surrounds them. The water-loving end of the detergent enables the dirt to be washed away since it is attracted to the water you splash on your face. The surfactant also helps water to be spread more easily on the skin.

You need a good cleanser to wash your face with. Water does not mix with oil, and cannot remove the oil from your skin without the help of a cleanser.

Soaps are commonly used as cleansers. They are formed by mixing fats or oils with an alkali substance (an alkali is the opposite of an acid). Because soaps are sometimes too drying to the skin, synthetic detergents, or syndets, are often used. These syndets are used in combination with other ingredients to give the product the characteristics you desire. So, ingredients to moisturize the skin, to help the cleanser lather more, to smell good, or to achieve the desired color are added to a detergent to make the final product. Other ingredients may be added to increase the stability of the formula, or to discourage bacterial growth. Anionic, or negatively charged, surfactants are

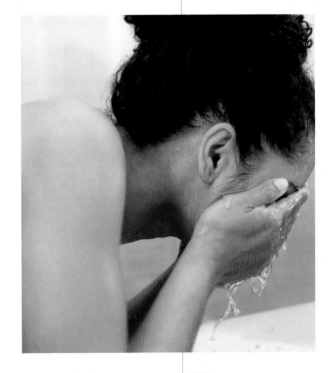

commonly used in skin care products. Sodium laurel sulfate is often used because, in addition to being a good cleanser, it has pleasing foaming qualities and is stable and easy to formulate. Sodium laureth sulfate and sodium sulphosuccinate are other ingredients you might see in your cleanser.

Anionic surfactants can be irritating to sensitive skin and should be avoided. Amphoteric surfactants are less irritating than anionics, and include sodium laurimino dipropionate and cocamido propyl betaine. Moisturizers such as glycerine or lanolin may be added to the cleanser. They give the most moisture after the skin has been washed.

> Even for the most sensitive skin, a cleanser is necessary because it enables you to clean your skin in a way that water alone cannot.

Cold creams are thick cleansers that include moisturizing ingredients. They are useful for cleansing dry skin and also for removing makeup. They are made of ingredients such as mineral oil or petrolatum. They are not appropriate for people with oily or acne-prone skin.

Exfoliators remove dead skin cells from the surface of the skin to reveal the more lustrous skin beneath. Exfoliating can be useful for people with dry skin and also for people with acne-prone skin because it can help to unblock the pores. One method of exfoliating uses chemicals to increase the rate of cell turnover and make the skin cells easier to remove. A second method uses a mechanical action to scrub away dead skin cells.

Chemical exfoliants include retinols, alpha-hydroxy acids such as glycolic acid and lactic acid, and beta-hydroxy acids such as salicylic acid.

These ingredients are found in many over-the-counter products. They are available in higher concentrations in products available through a

5 HOMEMADE EXFOLIATORS

- Make a paste using oatmeal and warm water to gently exfoliate dry or irritated skin.

- Mix equal parts of sea salt and an oil like almond oil, olive oil, or baby oil to make a coarse scrub for the body skin.

- Combine one teaspoon of baking soda or cornmeal in your favorite liquid facial cleanser for a mild weekly facial scrub.

- Add sugar to honey or oil for a gentle, skin-softening scrub.

- Coffee grounds can be mixed into the oil of your choice for a skin smoothing scrub.

dermatologist's office. Some of these agents are also used for chemical peels.

Mechanical exfoliants include natural products such as ground fruit pits or almond shells, sugar, or salt added to a cleanser. Other ingredients used are aluminum oxide crystals, like those used in microdermabrasion, or polyethalene beads. Pumice is used on the feet but is too rough for other parts of the body. Instead of looking for a product with an exfoliator in it, you can exfoliate by using any cleanser applied to a bath sponge, loofah, brushes, or microfiber cloth.

Toners are intended for use after cleansing and before moisturizing. They are meant to provide supplemental cleansing, and may provide additional attributes, such as moisturization or drying.

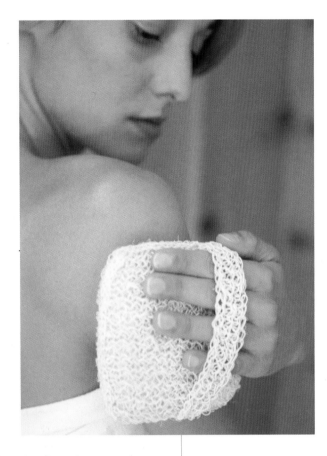

Gentle exfoliation helps to loosen and remove any dead skin cells on the surface of our skin.

Toners for oily skin contain alcohol, which removes any sebum or debris left behind by cleansing. If a toner is too strong, oily skin will be dry for a short time but will respond with a rebound oiliness within a few hours. Toners for dry skin do not contain alcohol. They may contain glycerine instead. Glycerine is a humectant, which holds water in and helps to moisturize the skin.

Step 2: Treating

At different times in your life, there will be areas of your facial skin that will require special attention. Whether you need to clear up a pimple, get rid

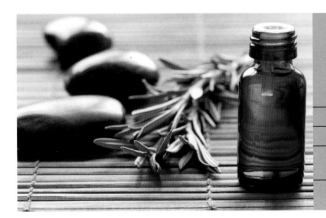

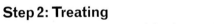

NATURAL TONERS

Several natural products make excellent toners. You may have these items around the house:

- **Witch hazel used alone**
- **Tea tree oil mixed with witch hazel**
- **Lemon juice diluted in water**
- **Rose petals steeped in boiling water and allowed to cool**
- **Apple cider vinegar diluted in water**

of a dark spot or reduce redness, applying products to address these special needs is usually best performed between cleansing and moisturizing so that the treatment comes directly in contact with the skin, and absorption is not delayed or reduced by the moisturizer.

Of course, the application of prescription medication for conditions like acne, rosacea, and seborrheic dermatitis on the face take precedence over the use of over-the-counter treatments.

Fade creams are used all over the world, by millions of individuals to lighten unwanted discoloration, even out the pigmentation of their skin, or just brighten the skin. Creams used to fade dark spots or even the complexion are known by many different names, among them fade creams, lightening creams, and evening creams. In some countries the term "whitening creams" is used, but in other countries this term is considered racially charged. In the United States, use of the term "bleaching cream" is limited to products containing hydroquinone.

Hydroquinone is a chemical that is effective in decreasing pigmentation in the skin. It has become a source of controversy in the cosmetic and medical communities in recent years. This is because some evidence indicates that hydroquinone may be carcinogenic in laboratory animals. It has not been shown to be carcinogenic in humans, though it has been in use for several decades. The main side-effect of hydroquinone in humans is a condition called exogenous ochronosis: an unwanted grey, brown, blue, or black pigmentation occurs in the skin, making it darker rather than lighter. The risk for ochronosis seems to be higher when higher concentrations of the product are used or when it is used for a long time. Hydroquinone is available in over-the-counter products in concentrations of up to 2 percent in the United States, but physicians can prescribe higher concentrations.

Because of the controversy surrounding hydroquinone, the cosmetics industry has searched for other ingredients effective in lightening the skin. Ingredients containing arbutin are widely used. Arbutin is found in the extracts of bearberry, mulberry, cranberry, and blueberry. Licorice extract contains glabridin, another effective ingredient. Vitamin C also reduces pigmentation, and alpha-hydroxy acids and retinoids increase the skin's cell turnover and reduce the time a dark spot is present. Mequinol is available as a prescription in combination with the retinoid tretinoin. Some ingredients are controversial. Glutathione is a common ingredient in skin

SKIN SOLUTION

While the use of hydroquinone is prohibited in some countries, several other skin fading ingredients are widely available in over-the-counter products, including arbutin, vitamin C, mulberry extract, and licorice extract.

The safety of hydroquinone is currently being debated within the medical community.

lightening products in some countries, but its effectiveness has not been demonstrated. Kojic acid is considered to be an effective ingredient. Its use in products is limited by concern about potential carcinogenicity and by challenges about its stability and like hydroquinone, it has been banned in some countries.

Skin serums are aimed at treating specific problems. They are characteristically light-weight liquids that contain active ingredients. The fact that they are not heavy allows you to layer on more than one serum to create a very customized skin care regimen, and makes them appropriate for use under your moisturizer or makeup. The active ingredient is usually a key selling point for these products since they are geared towards being effective and results-driven. Some serums serve to hydrate the skin. Others plump the skin to minimize the appearance of fine lines. Glycolic acid is one of the ingredients commonly found in exfoliating serums. Antioxidants are often found in antiaging serums. Collagen and peptides are other ingredients that are currently popular to add to these products.

Eye creams provide moisture to the delicate eyelid skin. There are creams available that claim to treat puffiness, dark circles and wrinkles. The truth of the matter is that some of these preparations provide better results than others, but there is truly no miracle cream. Eye creams contain many of the same ingredients that facial moisturizers do, but often in lower concentrations in order to minimize the risk of irritation. Common ingredients include antioxidants like vitamin C, exfoliants like glycolic acid, skin renewing substances like retinol and peptides.

Many people use hemorrhoid cream under the eyes to reduce under eye swelling. In fact, these creams can be very irritating to the eyelid skin and should only be used in their intended location.

Lip treatments can provide you with soft, kissable lips. How do you keep yours pucker-ready? Start by exfoliating. When you brush your teeth, gently brush your lips with your toothbrush to remove dead skin cells. Your lips are then ready for whatever product you choose. Most lip plumpers are really just mild irritants which cause blood flow to the lips to increase. You may also get a slight stinging sensation that accompanies application. Lip balms can help to seal in moisture, and some contain sunscreens to protect the lips from the sun.

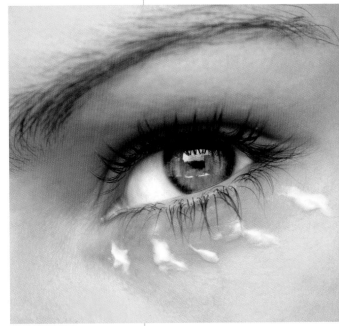

Step 3: Moisturizing

Moisturizers are used to keep the skin hydrated. It is important to apply your moisturizer

ANTIAGING IN A NUTSHELL

What are you willing to do in order to maintain your appearance? Some people want to stick to the basics, while others want to go all out. Here are the no-nonsense nuts and bolts of what works to slow or reverse the appearance of aging. Let your own desires, comfort level, and budget help you decide what is right for you:

Behavioral adjustments

- Protect your skin from the sun every day using hats, protective clothing, and sunscreen.
- Stop smoking; if you are not a smoker, don't start.
- Develop and maintain a daily routine that includes morning and evening skin care.

Proper nutrition

- Drink at least 4 pints (2 litres) of plain water every day.
- Eat a diet rich in antioxidants, including fruits like berries, grapes, and tomatoes and vegetables like broccoli, spinach, and carrots.
- Make sure that you are getting enough vitamin D from food sources, or take a supplement.

Over-the-counter skin care

- Find a gentle, effective cleanser that is not irritating.
- Treat skin problems promptly.
- Moisturize as needed.
- Wear sunscreen with UVA and UVB protection, at least SPF 30.

Prescription medication

- Retinoids including tretinoin, adapalene, and tazarotene are proven to improve the quality of the skin by thickening it, increasing collagen production, and smoothing the surface. Ask your doctor if a prescription is appropriate for you.

Youth-preserving medical procedures

- Chemical peels even the color of the skin and smooth its surface.
- Botox injections freeze the wrinkles that come from facial expression.
- Dermal fillers correct deep wrinkles.
- Laser treatments even the texture and color of the skin and can provide skin tightening.

Plastic surgery

- Blepharoplasty will give your eyes a rested, refreshed look.
- Face lift is still the gold standard for the most dramatic removal of wrinkles and sagging skin.

immediately after cleansing and treating the skin, while it is still damp. This maximizes the effectiveness of the moisturizer by "sealing" the water in the skin before it has a chance to evaporate. Three main types of ingredients are used in moisturizers.

Humectants attract water to the epidermis. This water may come from the dermis or from the environment.

Occlusive ingredients coat the skin to prevent moisture loss through evaporation, trapping water in the skin.

Emollients leave the skin feeling soft and smooth. Some ingredients serve more than one of these functions, and many commercially available moisturizers contain two or more moisturizing ingredients.

Cyclomethicone and dimethicone are used in products for people with oily skin because these products are silicone-based and thus are not oily. Ingredients used in heavier moisturizers for people with dry skin include mineral oil, petrolatum, and paraffin. Lanolin is used sometimes but may be irritating to sensitive skin. There are other effective ingredients that may be used in a moisturizer. These are just a few of the most common ones.

Step 4: Protection

It is vital to protect your skin from the harmful rays of sunlight. It is best to wear sunscreen every day, all year round to help reduce the development of wrinkles, blotchy skin discoloration, and most importantly, to decrease your risk of getting skin cancer.

Sunscreens provide protection from the effects of the sun's ultraviolet rays on the skin. These rays are categorized by their wavelength. Ultraviolet A (UVA) rays are longer and have wavelengths of 320–400 nm. Ultraviolet B (UVB) rays are shorter and have wavelengths of 290–320 nm. There are ultraviolet C rays, but they do not penetrate the ozone layer.

SKIN SOLUTION

You may need to change your moisturizer as the seasons change. A lighter lotion is appropriate for most people in warmer weather, whereas heavier creams may be necessary in cooler months.

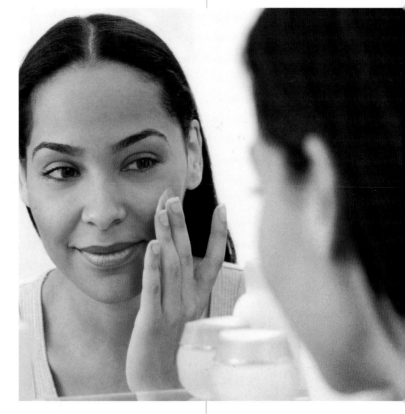

Apply moisturizer once or twice a day, depending on the specific needs of your skin.

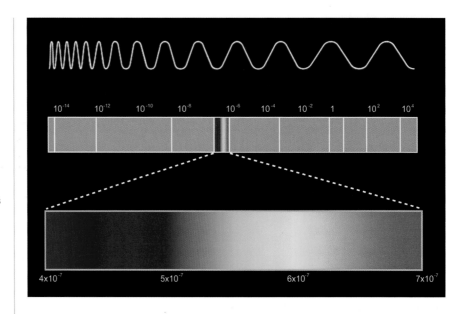

Visible light falls in the middle of the electromagnetic spectrum, with wavelengths from 380 to 750 nm. Shorter wavelengths (left) include gamma rays, X-rays, and ultraviolet light. Longer wavelengths (right) include infrared, microwaves, and radio waves.

The sun protection factor of a sunscreen gives an indication of how well a particular product protects you from UVB rays. The numerical value tells you how many times longer you can stay in the sunlight without burning compared to if your skin was unprotected. For instance, if you can normally stay in the sunlight for 10 minutes without burning, by putting on a sunscreen with an SPF of 30 you could stay in the sunlight for 300 minutes, or 5 hours, without burning. It is important to note that these values are determined in a controlled, laboratory setting. In real life, sunscreen needs to be reapplied every two hours and every time you get out of the water, even if it is waterproof.

Currently there is a rating system to measure protection from UVA rays. Most products recognize this feature as desirable and include their UVA protection on the label. Several ingredients provide effective protection against sunlight. Titanium dioxide and zinc oxide reflect and scatter the sun's rays away from the skin. They are sometimes referred to as "physical blockers." These ingredients protect against both UVA and UVB rays. They are particularly good ingredients for people with sensitive skin because they tend to be less irritating than some of the UV-absorbing sunscreens. The main disadvantage of these products is that they can leave the skin with a chalky appearance. Other ingredients work by absorbing the sun's rays. They are sometimes called "chemical blockers." Ingredients you can look for that absorb UVA rays include the following: avobenzone (parsol 1789), dioxybenzone (benzophenone-8), ecamsule (mexoryl), meradimate, which was formerly known as menthyl anthranilate (neo heliopan MA), and oxybenzone (neo heliopan bb).

Ingredients effective against UVB include paba, homosalate (hms), octyl methoxycinnamate (parsol mcx, escalol 557), octyl salicylate (escalol 587), padimate o (escalol 507), phenylbenzimidazole sulfonic acid (eusolex 232, parsol hs), and trolamine salicylate.

Ingredients effective against both UVA and UVB include octocylene escalol 597, cinoxate, and sulisobenzone (ums 40).

The proper application of sunscreen is essential regardless of the brand you choose. Sunscreen should be applied in an even layer over all of the skin's surface and must be reapplied every two hours. As mentioned previously, it also needs to be reapplied every time you get out of the water.

Your body skin type

We spend a lot of time thinking about the skin on our face. However, most of our skin exists from the neck down. The skin on the body has many of the same challenges that facial skin does. It needs to be cleaned and moisturized. It may be dry or prone to heavy perspiration. It may be sensitive to specific ingredients. Acne may occur on the chest, back, or even the buttocks. Dark spots may occur. And body skin also shows signs of aging. Many of the products marketed as body care products follow the same principles discussed above. In the following section, we discuss products that are predominantly for the body.

Cosmetic products for the body

There are now numerous products that we can apply to our skin for a wide variety of reasons—from preventing sweating, to tanning our skin, to treating concerns such as cellulite.

Deodorants and antiperspirants

Underarm perspiration is caused by secretions from the apocrine and the eccrine sweat glands. The amount of sweat produced is largely based on the body's efforts to regulate temperature. The higher the temperature, the more you perspire. This is how the body cools itself off.

Effective antiperspirants can be found in many forms, including aerosols, roll-ons, and solid and gel sticks.

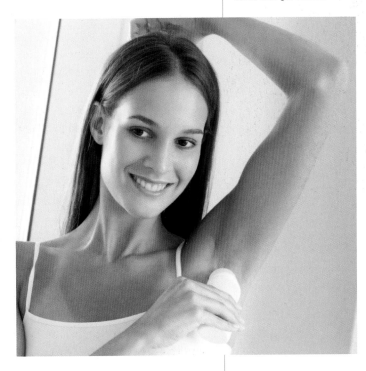

45

Have you ever noticed that you sweat more when you are nervous? That is because emotional factors also play a role in how much you perspire.

Perspiration itself does not have an unpleasant odor. However, it provides a very agreeable environment for the skin's normal bacteria to live and multiply. These bacteria break the sweat down into fatty acids that have the characteristic unpleasant odor. The hair under the arms provides additional surfaces for both the bacteria and the sweat to reside, so the more hair you have under your arms, the more sweat and odor you will have.

Two types of products are useful for managing perspiration. Deodorants mask or reduce the odor associated with sweat. Antiperspirants reduce the amount of sweat produced by blocking the sweat glands. Many commercially available products have ingredients that deal with the amount of perspiration and the odor, making them both antiperspirants and deodorants.

In order to understand how a product works, look at the ingredients. Deodorants contain perfumes that are more pleasant than the odor of sweat. On an ingredient list, these will apprear as "fragrance." They may also contain ingredients such as triclosan, triclocarbon, benzethonium chloride, or chlorhexidine. These ingredients have antibiotic properties and reduce the amount of bacteria on the skin. Less bacteria means less free fatty acid production and less odor.

Metal salts are used as antiperspirants. They block the opening of the sweat gland so that less perspiration is released. Metal salts commonly used include aluminum chloride, aluminum chlorohydrate, aluminum dichlorohydrate, aluminum sesquichlorohydrate, aluminum zirconium chlorohydrate, and buffered aluminum sulfate. These ingredients are listed as the active ingredients on the product label.

Many people have sensitive skin under the arms and require a special deodorant. You may be allergic to the fragrance and require a fragrance-free product. Or you might try one of the antiperspirant stones. They are made of mineral salts that contain an ingredient called alum. Most users notice that these products reduce sweating and odor and also cause less irritation than traditional products.

Make sure that you exfoliate before applying a self-tanning product to ensure smooth and even coverage.

Sunless tanners

Many people use sunscreens to protect the skin from the sunlight, but some still like the look of tanned skin. There are safe and effective ways to achieve a tanned appearance without increasing your risk of skin cancer or prematurely aging your skin.

Bronzers are cosmetic products that contain brown pigments. They are usually purchased as a powder or a lotion. The product is applied to the skin and instantly imparts a tanned look. These products wash off, and no residual color is left behind.

Self-tanners contain an ingredient called dihydroxyacetone (DHA). This is a type of sugar that reacts with the keratins in the stratum corneum, the uppermost layer of the skin. This reaction forms melanoidin, a brown pigmentation that is different from the skin's natural melanin. This pigmentation does not simply wash off. It is removed as the stratum corneum cells slough off, or desquamate. The tan color from DHA generally lasts for about five to seven days. Most products are reapplied every three days to maintain the tan appearance.

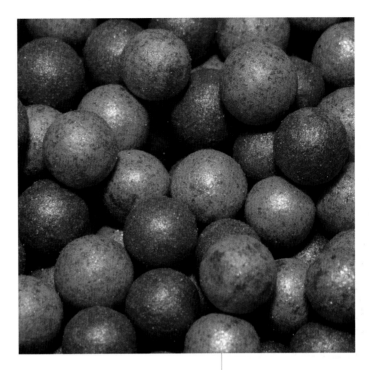

Bronzers are a safe and simple way to give your skin a natural and healthy color, without any risks.

Like melanin, the melanoids formed by DHA provide some protection from the sun. Skin tanned using self-tanners has an SPF of approximately 3. This is not adequate sun protection, so sunscreens should be used even if you have darkened your skin with a self-tanning product.

Both cosmetics containing bronzers and self-tanners containing DHA are considered to be safe by both the dermatology community and the U.S. Food and Drug Administration. Dermatologists often recommend both types of product as an alternative to tanning.

There are two main ingredients in tanning pills: carotenoids and tyrosine. Carotenoids, orange pigments, are found in nature. They are the substance that gives carrots their color. Several carotenoids are used in tanning pills, including canthaxanthin, beta carotene, and lycopene. Canthaxanthin is used in small amounts as a food colorant and is considered safe by the U.S. FDA for this use. It must be taken in much larger doses to impart color to skin. These doses have been associated with liver damage, eye problems, and hives. Tanning pills containing this ingredient are not approved by the U.S. FDA and are sometimes blocked from entry into the United States.

Tanning pills containing tyrosine are sometimes called tan accelerators. Tyrosine is an amino acid found naturally in the body. Although some

SKIN SOLUTION

Despite restrictive regulations in several countries, tanning pills are widely available for purchase on the Internet. It is important to note that no tanning pills are approved by the United States FDA. However, self-tanners are a safe way to achieve tanned looking skin.

products claim that these pills increase melanin synthesis, there is no good scientific evidence to support this claim. But there is evidence that it is not effective.

The safest way to achieve a tanned appearance is through the use of temporary bronzer products or self-tanners containing DHA that are topically applied. Tanning pills are not approved by the U.S. FDA and are not recommended by most doctors.

Cellulite creams

Dimples on the face are considered attractive. Dimples on the thighs and buttocks are not. Cellulite is very common in women and is sometimes seen in men, too. It is a result of deposits of fat under the skin, pushing on the connective tissue that supports the skin, and forms bulges. Genes, weight, age, and skin thickness all play a role in the appearance of cellulite.

Some of us have learned to embrace cellulite as part of our skin. Others search for a solution with the same fervor that Ponce de León displayed in searching for the Fountain of Youth. Because of the large demand for a treatment, many different cellulite creams with a variety of active ingredients are available. No cream provides a cure for cellulite, and there is some debate over the ability of cellulite creams to improve the condition. And although some active ingredients have effects on the skin that may be theoretically helpful, some scientists dispute the actual effectiveness of these creams with those active ingredients. However, many consumers use these products routinely and perceive a benefit.

What ingredients should you look for? Different ingredients work in different ways, and some products contain multiple anti-cellulite ingredients. Caffeine and aminophylline, both commonly used, decrease the fluid content of the skin. Some ingredients, such as L-carnitine and bupleurun falcatum, help the body to break down the fat. Green tea is thought to stimulate the release of stored fat.

Retinols help to encourage skin cell turnover, improving the appearance of the skin. Peptides stimulate collagen production to improve the firmness of the skin. The good news is that all of these products are safe to try. And the mechanical action of massaging creams into lumpy areas twice a day may contribute to improving the appearance of the skin.

Skin Myth

True or False?

If you have cellulite you must be overweight.

False

Genetic factors, skin thickness, and age all play a role in the development of cellulite. People who are slim can develop cellulite just as overweight people can.

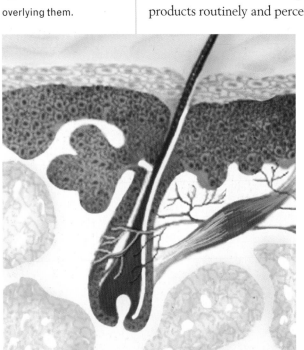

Cellulite appears when subcutaneous fat cells give a dimpled appearance to the skin overlying them.

Common facial concerns

Out of all the areas of the body, women are most concerned with the appearance of their face. It is the part of the body that we present first to the world. Our faces reflect our beauty, identity, and vitality. We strive for clear, even-toned skin, free of discolorations, dullness, and redness.

Everyone would like their facial skin to be flawless, but there will always be an unwelcome lump, bump, spot, or mark. These unwanted growths may turn out to be cysts, moles (nevi), enlarged oil glands (sebaceous hyperplasia), or benign papules (dermatosis papulosa nigra). Additionally, pores may appear too large and undereye circles may be too dark. Simple maneuvers, such as regular exfoliation may aid in reducing the appearance of pores and skin brighteners may reduce dark undereye circles.

Most of us feel the temptation to pick or squeeze facial lumps and bumps. Resist the urge as this can lead to scarring.

If there are growths on the skin that don't go away, any new or changing growth must be checked by your doctor to ensure that it is not cancerous or pre-cancerous. This is very important. In fact, you should have a head-to-toe, total body skin examination every year by a dermatologist. Let them know if any growth has changed in size, shape, or color.

Although manipulating the lumps, bumps, or spots make us feel that we are improving the situation, we are harming the skin and making it susceptible to infections and scars. Remember that most growths can be removed safely by your doctor, so keep your hands off them. With just a little knowledge and the appropriate treatment, our dissatisfaction with our facial skin will disappear.

Squeezing or manipulating either an epidermoid cyst or a pimple can lead to infection or scarring of the skin.

Acne

Acne can be a nuisance from the teen years all the way into the forties and over. Deeper cystic lesions can even be painful. Not only are the pimples annoying, they can leave pink or dark spots that last for several weeks, and ice-pick scars from acne are permanent. See Chapter 3 for a detailed discussion of acne and the treatment options.

Cysts

Cysts can occur anywhere on the body, but often they don't bother people unless they occur on the face. If you have noticed a firm, round lump under the surface of your skin, or

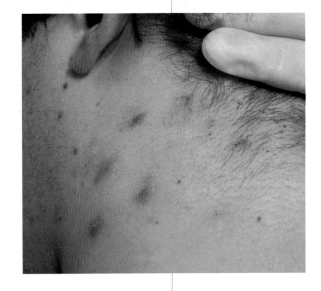

THE ABCDE's OF EVALUATING MOLES

- **A** Asymmetry
- **B** Border
- **C** Color
- **D** Diameter
- **E** Evolving

one that protrudes above the skin's surface and does not go away, it is most likely to be an epidermoid cyst. An epidermoid cyst is filled with a material called keratin that has a unique and unpleasant odor. Cysts can increase or decrease in size, depending upon how much keratin is in the cyst, and sometimes a cottage cheese like substance is expressed from a central pore.

As long as you do not squeeze this type of lump, you will not have a problem and treatment will be effective. Squeezing could cause inflammation and the development of an infection.

If you do not like the appearance of an epidermoid cyst, it can be treated in one of three ways:

1. The cyst can be cut and the keratin drained from it (I & D)
2. It can be injected with a cortisone medication to cause it to shrink
3. It can be cut out and the skin closed with stitches

The first two methods are the least invasive, but the cyst could recur. Total removal of the cyst will prevent recurrence, but the procedure will cause a permanent scar.

Nevi (moles)

The most common type of "bump" found on the face is a mole, or nevus. Moles occur on the forehead, cheeks, nose, and chin; and depending upon your skin tone, they may be skin-colored, pink, tan, brown, black, or blue. Individuals with darker skin tones tend to have darker moles, so someone of East Indian descent will, in general, have very dark moles compared to someone of northern European descent. Moles may be raised or flat, and can even begin flat and become raised in time. In the United States, flat, dark facial moles have been referred to as beauty marks, and both Marilyn Monroe and Cindy Crawford have been admired for their distinctive beauty marks. In contrast, these marks are not considered symbols of beauty in Japan.

Most moles are benign and no treatment is required. It is easy to determine if your mole is benign by following the ABCDE rules (see chapter 1). Moles can be removed for cosmetic reasons by a dermatologist or plastic surgeon using surgical scissors or a blade. The results are usually very good, although scarring is a potential side-effect. Moles should not be burned off with an electric needle or removed with a laser because a portion of the mole may remain and could lead to undetected skin cancer. If you have any questions about a mole, they should be examined by your doctor.

Enlarged pores

Pores are more than just tiny holes in the skin. They are the opening of a hair follicle that allows not only the hair but also oil to reach the surface of the skin. Each person's pore size is slightly different. They may appear larger in those with oily skin. Pores are lined with skin cells that are shed daily. They sometimes get clogged when they fill with debris from dead skin cells and trapped sebum. This causes the pores to appear larger than normal and may form a bump on the skin called a closed comedone or whitehead. If the debris in the pore gets exposed to oxygen in the air through a pore that is sufficiently distended, the material turns black. The bump is then called an open comedone, or a blackhead. Blackheads and whiteheads occur in acne-prone skin.

Topical creams as well as physical, manual, or chemical exfoliation to remove dead skin cells and debris from pores can all improve pore appearance and size. Physical extractions of pores to release and remove the plug and dead cells can be performed by an esthetician or doctor using an instrument called a comedone extractor. It is important that this procedure is done gently and by a professional so as not to damage the skin or cause a worsening of acne. Often the skin is pretreated with medicated cream to loosen the plug before physical exfoliation is performed.

Creams containing ingredients such as the alpha hydroxy acids (AHAs) and the glycolic, citric, lactic, malic, and tartaric acids; the prescription retinoids tretinoin, retin A, adapalene, or tazaratene, or non-prescription retinol; or the beta hydroxy acid (BHA) salicylic acid can accelerate the removal of dead skin cells and also remove plugs. Finally, chemical exfoliation with AHA or BHA chemical peels or microdermabrasion will help to improve pore appearance.

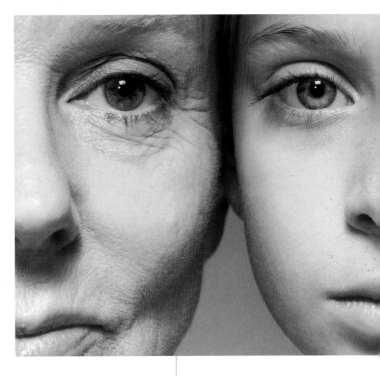

Pore size is determined by genetic factors and cannot be changed.

Redness

Facial redness is a common complaint, particularly in individuals with very pale or light skin tones. Redness can be caused by several factors. When skin is irritated by skin care products, topical medications, or harsh weather, it will become red. Redness also occurs when blood vessels open (dilate) and the flow of blood to the surface of the skin increases. The growth of thin blood vessels, telangiectasias, on the skin's surface will likewise cause redness. Certain skin diseases, such as rosacea and lupus, can cause redness of facial skin. People with darker skin tones may also experience facial redness, but this is often difficult to see clearly because melanin pigment may mask the redness. Rosacea and lupus are discussed further in chapter 3.

Pores do not have muscles and so cannot open and close. They can, however, get clogged with dirt so gentle cleansing is important.

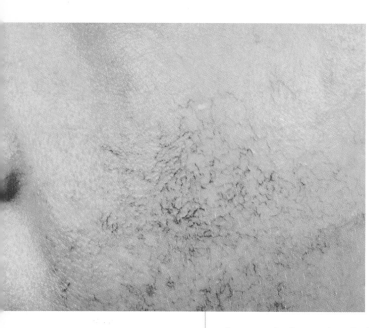

Facial redness can be an embarrassing problem for its sufferers.

Your first step in reducing facial redness is to use gentle skin care products. Look for non-irritating ingredients and ingredients that can help soothe the skin, such as green or white tea, licorice, or feverfew. You probably want to avoid products containing AHA and BHA and those containing retinoids. It is also important to cleanse your skin gently twice daily using only your fingertips and patting the skin dry with a soft, cotton towel. Always avoid rubbing the skin which will increase redness. If you are using topical medications that cause your skin to become red, discuss substitutions with your doctor. Several procedures can be performed by your doctor to lessen redness caused by telangiectasias. They may be burned with the electric needle (electrocautery), or treated with the pulsed dye laser (specific for blood vessels) or the intense pulsed light (IPL).

These procedures may be expensive and time-consuming, and a fast, inexpensive alternative is to simply camouflage the redness with a good concealer. Select a concealer that contains a green tint effective in neutralizing the red color. Then your foundation can be applied over the concealer and the redness will disappear. If you need help in selecting the right makeup, ask for advice from the staff at the beauty counter.

SKIN SOLUTION

If you have a lot of facial discoloration, try using camouflage makeup instead of regular makeup to hide the imperfections. It provides better coverage and lasts longer. Just be sure to use a good makeup remover at the end of the day.

Dull skin tones

We all strive for radiant and glowing facial skin. However, dull skin tone may occur at various times of the year, caused by dry, cold winter weather or by too much sun, sand, and surf in the summer. Dull skin tone also occurs in the late 30s, the 40s, and beyond because skin cells become sticky and are not properly shed. The key to restoring radiant skin is exfoliation. Exfoliation may be achieved manually with abrasive beads, kernels, sugars, or salts in topical scrubs. Loofah-type sponges or puffs are a manual way to exfoliate superficial skin cells. Microdermabrasion, performed by a health care professional, utilizes crystals or a diamond tip to gently sand away the dull layers of skin. Lastly, chemical peels utilizing various chemicals such as glycolic acid, salicylic acid, or trichloracetic acid are effective in skilled hands. Individuals with darker skin tones must be aware that some abrasives and peels may irritate their skin and produce dark marks or discoloration. You should let your doctor know if you experience discomfort during a microdermabrasion or chemical peel.

Hyperpigmentation

Excessive pigmentation can occur in all skin types, but it is a particular problem for people with darker skin tones, such as those of Asian, African, Latin, or Native American backgrounds. Melanin is the chemical that determines the color of skin. The more melanin there is in a person's skin, the darker that person's skin will be. Sometimes the cells that produce melanin are damaged or over-stimulated. A rash, acne, pimple, or even sunburn can cause these cells to go into overdrive. When this happens, the affected cells may begin to produce too much melanin. Too much melanin causes darker spots or patches.

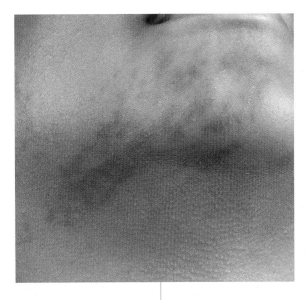

Dark marks on the skin may last for months or even years after they develop. Sun protection and swift treatment allow them to fade much faster.

Treatment of hyperpigmentation begins with protecting the skin from the stimulating ultraviolet rays of the sun. Applying a sunscreen of SPF 30 or higher daily is essential to treatment. You should also avoid the sun by walking on the shady side of the street, wear a wide-brimmed hat or large sunglasses to help protect your skin from the sun.

Topical medications containing ingredients such as hydroquinone, azelaic acid, kojic acid, bearberry, licorice, and retinoid are also helpful in treating darker patches, as are chemical peels and microdermabrasion.

Dark under-eye circles

People might ask if you are tired, but there are other reasons that you may have dark circles under your eyes. One common cause is poor drainage of blood from the veins under the eyes into the veins of the nose. This can occur whenever there is nasal congestion, like if you have seasonal allergies. Although dark circles can occur in all skin types, those with darker skin tones, especially African Americans, Southeast Asians, and Europeans of Mediterranean descent, are particularly troubled by hereditary dark circles. Additionally, as we age, the skin begins to thin and the lower eyelid skin appears darker.

Rinse used black or chamomile teabags with cold water and place on the eyelids for 10 minutes to reduce puffiness.

Treatment is aimed at plumping or thickening the lower eyelid skin and lightening the discolorations. Retinoids or AHAs (alpha hydroxy acid) may plump the skin by stimulating the production of collagen. Agents used to minimize or decrease pigmentation include vitamin K cream, kojic acid, and the antioxidant vitamin C.

Common body concerns

You may have one or more areas on your skin that you would like to change. It might be dark elbows or rough skin on the soles of the feet. While these cosmetic concerns will not affect your health, they may affect how you feel about yourself. The good news is that with a little extra attention and the right treatment, many problem areas can be a thing of the past.

Always remember that rubbing and scrubbing the skin will not improve your problems areas. In fact, vigorous washing may actually worsen several problems. Instead, always clean the skin very gently, rinse, and pat dry.

Dark elbows and knees

Dark elbows and knees are a common problem in both children and adults. Friction and pressure to skin of these areas and can lead to unwanted discolorations and may cause the skin to thicken as well. Think about how many times you lean on your elbows or kneel on your knees. Do you find yourself inadvertently rubbing, scratching, or scrubbing these areas? If the answer is yes, then you are likely contributing to the cause of the discoloration. In addition to brown discoloration, your elbow and knee skin may become thickened and rough to the touch. This often leads to us scrubbing the elbow and knee skin or using abrasive puffs or sponges while washing. But scrubbing or vigorous washing can actually worsen the darkness and thickness of the skin.

The first step in treating dark elbows and knees is gentle skin care. Throw out the harsh and abrasive agents that you are using on these areas. It is also important to minimize friction and injury to these areas, so your days of leaning on your elbows and kneeling on your knees are over.

Selecting the correct topical medication is the key to soft, smooth, even-colored elbows and knees. Although many people will tell you that lemon juice, cocoa butter, or green tea will help, there is no evidence to prove the effectiveness of these home remedies. Skin lightening creams are very effective,

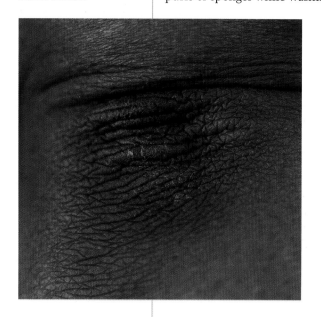

Leaning on your elbows repeatedly can cause the skin to darken.

and in North America the majority of skin-lightening creams contain hydroquinone. In Europe and Asia, where hydroquinone is not allowed, skin-lightening creams often include ingredients such as kojic acid, arbutin, or licorice. In addition to a skin-lightening cream, an exfoliating lotion containing ammonium lactate, urea, or salicylic acid will help remove the thickened rough skin and allow for better penetration of the lightening cream. These lotions should be applied once or twice every day. Finally, be patient. With most skin problems that you begin treating, results are seen in four to eight weeks.

Rough feet

Rough skin can occur on any part of your body, but it is a particular problem on the soles of the feet. The feet can even flake, peel, or crack and become painful. Rough feet occur in a variety of situations: walking barefoot, the constant rubbing of the feet by tight shoes, dry weather, and even fungal foot infections. This condition can be embarrassing when summer sandals reveal rough heels.

To remove the rough skin and restore smooth, soft feet, you want to exfoliate and hydrate the skin. Although the skin of the soles of the feet is the thickest skin on the entire body, it can become irritated and painful if the exfoliation is too vigorous. Exfoliation can be achieved by either abrasive or non-abrasive agents. Abrasive agents in foot creams may include ingredients such as salt, sugar, pits, seeds, or kernels. Rough sponges or puffs and pumice stones are also effective in removing thickened skin. Think of a pumice stone as sandpaper for your feet. It is important to introduce abrasive agents slowly and use them gently to avoid irritation and pain. For example gently rubbing a pumice stone on the soles of the feet for a few minutes each day will lead to softer feet after two weeks or so. Non-abrasive exfoliators contain ingredients such as salicylic acid and urea that are also effective in removing rough skin. Applying non-abrasive exfoliators to the skin once a day for several weeks will reveal the soft skin underneath. Don't apply non-abrasive exfoliating creams or lotions to broken or cracked skin, because they will sting or burn.

Dry skin on the feet can become rough and thickened and painful cracks or fissures may develop.

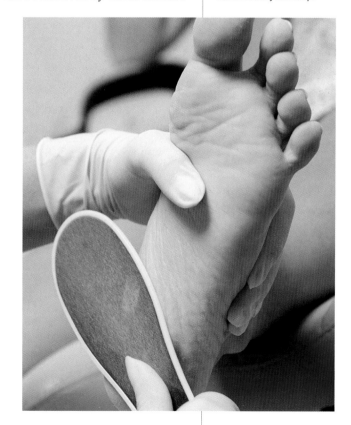

Moisturizing and hydrating the feet is also important for dealing with rough skin. A rich moisturizer, or something inexpensive such as white petroleum jelly (Vaseline), massaged onto the feet twice daily will be helpful. Consider wrapping the feet in plastic wrap (cling film) or covering them with plastic bags overnight. Alternatively, you can cover your feet with white cotton socks. Just a little extra time and attention can lead to soft, smooth feet.

Stretch marks first appear in adolescence when young people experience rapid growth spurts. These marks are unavoidable.

While retinoid creams are effective for treating stretch marks they cannot be used during pregnancy. If you are pregnant, use moisturizers on your abdomen until after delivery.

Stretch marks

Think about an elastic band or rubber band that you stretch too far and it breaks. Once the elastic band is broken, you cannot put it back together. The skin works the same way. Stretch marks (striae distensae) occur when the skin is quickly distended or stretched more than it should be and the skin's elastic fibers break. There is also a loss of the skin's collagen fibers that results in the thinning of the skin in the stretch mark. Stretch marks often occur on the abdomen after pregnancy, on the buttocks, breasts, or legs after a rapid weight gain or loss, and on the arms after weight-lifting causes muscles to bulge. The old saying that "an ounce of prevention is worth a pound of cure" is important in the case of stretch marks. Preventing some of them is possible simply by maintaining your normal weight and not overdoing it with muscle-building

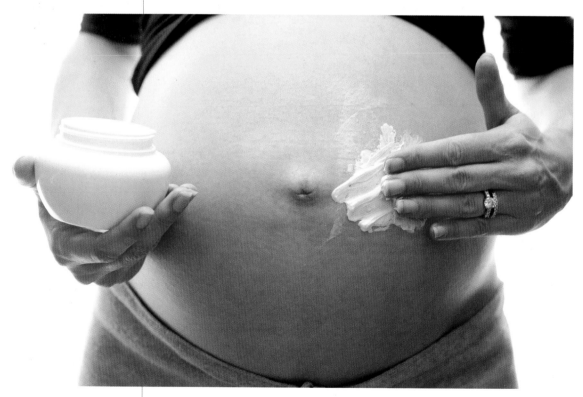

work-outs. Stretch marks may first appear as red or dark simply by maintaining your normal weight and not overdoing it with weights.

Stretch marks may first appear as red or dark brown lines on the skin that become lighter in color or even silvery as time goes by. Because the elastic fibers have been broken and collagen has been lost, it is impossible to make stretch marks disappear entirely. However, there are treatments that can improve their appearance. The best results occur when the marks have recently formed, and are red or brown.

There are many topical creams and lotions available in stores, on-line, and on television that promise to improve stretch marks, but beware. The only creams proven to be helpful are those that contain a form of vitamin A called tretinoin (Retin A). It has been shown that tretinoin cream (in a concentration of 0.1 percent) applied nightly, directly to the stretch mark improved the appearance of new stretch

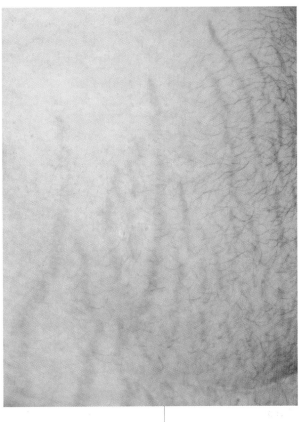

Stretch marks are pink or red when they first appear, but they become lighter over time.

marks by increasing the production of collagen and elastin in the skin and reducing the redness or darkness.

Another effective combination is using creams containing 20 percent glycolic acid applied in the morning, with either 0.05 percent tretinoin cream or 10 percent L-ascorbic acid (vitamin C) serum applied at night. This has shown to improve the appearance of light-colored stretch marks. When doctors looked at skin under the microscope, they found that skin treated with tretinoin formed new elastic fibers.

Side effects from tretinoin may occur and could include skin irritation, dryness, peeling, redness, or blistering of the skin. Individuals with darker skin must be particularly cautious because irritation could lead to long-lasting skin discoloration. In many countries, including the United States and Canada, tretinoin is only available by prescription.

Laser treatments with the pulse dye laser may be helpful to some people in reducing the depth of the stretch mark. Usually one treatment is required for stretch marks and it typically takes 15 minutes. Discomfort or pain during the treatment is mild. Improvement can be seen shortly after healing, and studies have demonstrated continued improvement in the appearance

SKIN SOLUTION

While stretch marks can't be erased completely, their appearance can be improved. Combining laser treatments with chemical peels or microdermabrasion is often the best treatment, but prescription creams offer a less pricey alternative.

of stretch marks up to 12 months after treatment. It appears that the laser increases the number of elastic fibers in the skin.

Laser treatments may be very expensive, and the results cannot be guaranteed. Treatments should be administered only by a certified dermatologist, plastic surgeon, or by one of their staff under their supervision. Individuals with darker skin types must exercise caution, and only seek treatment from doctors experienced in working with your skin type. Side effects such as permanent skin discoloration and bruising may occur. It is always a good practice to have a laser test spot performed on a small area of skin first. After you observe how the area has healed and you are happy with the results, then you can proceed with the full treatment.

> Laser treatments should not be performed on suntanned skin because burning and discoloration may occur. It is important to wait until after your suntan has faded before beginning laser treatments.

Seborrheic keratoses

Seborrheic keratoses are the most common benign tumor in older individuals. They occur in people of all racial groups and are pink, tan, or brown, depending upon one's skin tone. Although the cause is unknown, there is often a hereditary predisposition. Seborrheic keratoses have a stuck-on appearance and a rough surface resembling broccoli or cauliflower. They can appear at any place on the body and commonly occur on the trunk and the head. Seborrheic keratoses are about ⅛ to ¼ inch (½ to 1 cm) in size but can increase to 1 inch (2½ cm) in size or larger. They have no cancerous potential and are often regarded as a nuisance. Once irritated or inflamed, they may fall off spontaneously.

Treatment of seborrheic keratoses is unnecessary as the lesions are benign. However, many people want them removed for cosmetic reasons. This can be achieved with scissors or by shaving after the base of the lesion is numbed.

Hyperhidrosis

If your palms sweat profusely, especially when you are nervous, or if you ruin your clothing because of underarm sweating, then you probably have hyperhidrosis.

Located within the dermis are coiled sweat glands (green), sensory nerves (also green), and blood vessels (red and blue).

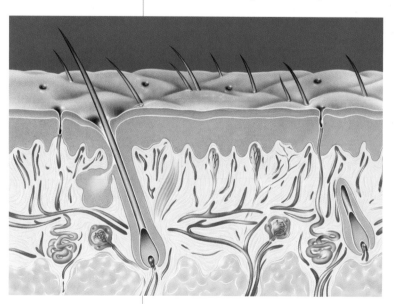

Hyperhidrosis is defined as at least one episode of excessive sweating per week for more than six months. Areas affected are the underarms, face, palms, and soles of the feet, and the episodes stop while you are asleep. Some people only sweat profusely in their sleep. These episodes are called night sweats. The most difficult aspect of hyperhidrosis is that it impairs your daily activities, preventing you from wanting to shake hands, to exercise, or to participate in certain social activities. It can also lead to difficulty in the normal activities of life such as handling paper, holding glasses or other slippery objects, or playing an instrument. Its impact on your life can range from the annoying (having to change your clothing or shoes frequently) to the dangerous (an electrical shock). Factors that may trigger excessive sweating include stress, anxiety, and social situations and also environmental factors such as heat and humidity.

Most people with hyperhidrosis have other family members with the disorder. Most sufferers are healthy with no underlying illness, and they are considered to have primary hyperhidrosis. Although most cases of hyperhidrosis are felt to result from overactivity of the nervous system, that causes the eccrine sweat glands to produce too much sweat, they can also be associated with more serious illnesses. The more serious form of hyperhidrosis, called secondary hyperhidrosis, may be due to an illness with a high fever, a spinal cord injury, diabetes, substance abuse, an infection, cancer, or even disorders of the heart, lung, or brain.

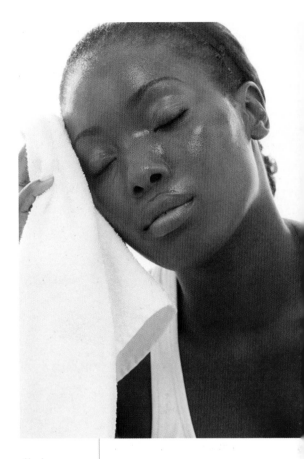

Profuse sweating is normal after strenuous exercise. It is how your body cools itself off.

Fortunately there are several effective treatments for hyperhidrosis, depending upon the severity of the condition. Treatment usually begins with topical prescription antiperspirants such as aluminum chloride hexahydrate, which is applied at bedtime to the affected area. These products work by blocking sweat ducts so that sweat does not reach the surface of the skin. In some people, aluminum chloride hexahydrate can lead to irritation, stinging, or burning of the skin. Using it at bedtime and washing it off the next morning can minimize irritation.

Treatment of excessive sweating has improved over the past several years so that you no longer have to suffer with this problem.

Iontophoresis is also used to treat hyperhidrosis. It is a process in which an electric current is delivered to the affected area to block the sweat ducts. The hands or feet are placed on a metal plate and a current is delivered for approximately 30 minutes, 4 to 5 days each week. An improvement may be observed after 5 to 10 treatments. Potential side effects may include irritation, dryness, or skin peeling. If topical agents are not effective in controlling sweating, injections of botulinum toxin into the underarm area, palms, or soles of the feet can dramatically decrease sweating; and the results can last for up to 9 months. It works by blocking the release of sweat from the glands. In the doctor's office, botulinum toxin is injected into the affected area with a small needle. The entire process takes about 20 minutes, with results seen as early as one week after injection. Although the procedure may be uncomfortable or painful, numbing medication can be used to make you more comfortable. Although uncommon, side effects may include bruising, tenderness, or loss of strength in the hands if the palms are injected.

Surgical treatments for hyperhidrosis are used when the less invasive treatments are not effective. Surgery targets the nerves of the sympathetic ganglia that stimulate the sweat glands to produce sweat. The nerves may be cut, clamped, or burned to relieve sweating in the palms, face, soles of the feet, and underarms. Although this treatment is effective, serious side effects have been reported. The possibility of such side effects needs to be discussed with the doctor.

Body odor

Hyperhidrosis means excessive sweating, but do you know what bromhidrosis means? You may have guessed that it means body odor. The apocrine sweat glands produce an odorless substance that is broken down by bacteria on the surface of the skin. This releases chemicals that produce an unpleasant odor, known as body odor. Everyone has body odor, and it is only a cause for concern if the odor changes dramatically, which may signal an internal illness.

The areas of the body that produce the strongest odor have the greatest number of apocrine glands. These are the underarm and genital areas. Our sensitivity to body odor differs depending upon our culture and accepted hygiene habits. Your diet, gender, genetics, general health, and the medication you take also influence your body odor. People of East Asian descent tend to have fewer sweat glands than people from that of other ethnic groups and hence they experience less sweating and body odor.

The treatment of body odor begins with good daily hygiene by washing with a cleanser and water to remove the perspiration as well as the bacteria on the skin. Deodorant soaps may be helpful, particularly during the summer months, in reducing odor. Shaving body hair will reduce sweating and bacteria. Antiperspirants help to decrease perspiration. Clothing is a

---

Skin Myth

True or False?

Body odor begins in adolescence because the bathing habits of teens are poor.

False

In fact, body odor begins at puberty because that is when the apocrine sweat glands of the under arms and genital region start to produce their secretions.

Hidrosis is the Greek word for sweating. Bromhidrosis is sweating that produces body odor, chromhidrosis is the production of colored sweat, and hyperhidrosis is excessive perspiration. All three can be a major annoyance.

reservoir of odors from the body, so do not forget to wash or dry-clean your clothes on a regular basis.

Body accessories

Using accessories to adorn our bodies can be fun and whimsical or a statement of an important ideal or principle. It is a representation of who we are and allows us to express ourselves in a variety of ways. Body accessories are not limited to clothing, shoes, hats, belts and the like, but we can accessorize our skin with body piercings and tattoos. Whereas the henna tattoos in the hands of Indian women that symbolize weddings and marriage are temporary and fade away over time, ink tattoos should be considered permanent. Although many tattoos can be removed with surgery or laser treatment, it is a time consuming and expensive process. The holes produced by body piercings will close with time but a mark may remain. The bottom line is to think carefully and make sure that the body accessory that you get today will be acceptable and pleasing to you in 10 or 20 years. There is little point in enduring the process of a piercing or tattoo only to regret it later. Remember also to think beyond pure beauty and consider if the area is prone to infection, or if the piercing can affect your ability to continue your regular activities after you have been pierced.

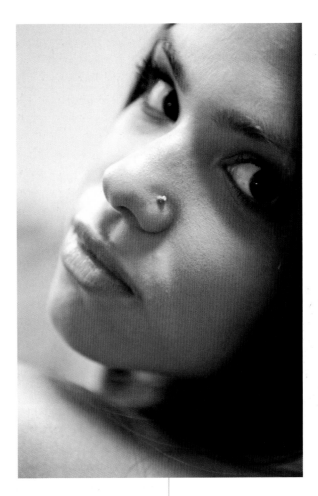

Discuss the proper care of your piercing with the person who performs the procedure in order to prevent side effects like infection and scarring.

Body piercing

Body piercing is a unique way to decorate your body and to express your individuality. It is practiced on just about every continent. Piercing is popular on the ears, nose, tongue, belly button, chest, and genital areas. It should always be performed by a professional in clean conditions, with the piercer wearing new gloves. The area of your body to be pierced should be disinfected with alcohol before piercing, and only sterile needles or disposable needles should be used on any area other than the earlobe. During the actual piercing, the piercer will pass a hollow needle through the chosen body part, which will create a tunnel. This usually feels like a prick or sting. The body jewelry is inserted in the tunnel. A small amount of bleeding may occur as a result of the piercing. To minimize bleeding discuss with your

Location of piercing	General information
Ear lobes - non cartilage	The lobe is the easiest place on the body to pierce and has the highest success rate. It generally heals well, and accommodates many different styles of jewelry. However, ear lobes are the most common sites for keloids to develop. A lobe piercing can also be stretched.
Lobe orbital	A rare piercing performed only by a very experienced, professional piercer. Jewelry will hang side to side through the lobe, rather than from front to back.
Helix	Piercing through the curled (cartilage) ridge on the outer edge of the ear. May be painful and slower to heal.
Helix orbital and antihelix	Piercing of two holes required rather than one. Jewelry is placed from side to side rather than front to back or it may "orbit" the helix like rings around a planet.
Rook	Piercing above the tragus (cartilage). Technically difficult depending on the thickness of the tragus and requires an experienced professional. Infection more likely.

Location of piercing	General information
Daith	Piercing above the tragus through a thick section of cartilage. Requires longer healing process, as a larger wound is created. Infection more likely.
Tragus	Piercing the thick layer of cartilage just below the rook. Technically more difficult. Infection possible.
Industrial	Piercings that are connected with an extra long barbell.
Conch	Also called a "shell" for the way this part of the ear resembles a seashell. As with all cartilage piercings, will be subject to soreness and infection.
Conch orbital	Piercing runs perpendicular to the regular conch piercing, which requires 2 holes allowing the ring to "orbit" the ear's cartilage.

BODY PIERCINGS

Location of piercing	General information
Eyebrow	Piercing along the brow line. Meticulous care required to avoid risk of infection.
Bridge	Piercing horizontally across the bridge of the nose, on the skin surface. Migration possible and technically difficult.
Above lip (Beauty mark)	Piercing is through the outside of the lip area. Also called the "Monroe" or "Madonna," this piercing simulates a beauty mark.
Tongue	Piercings are done at the front of the tongue. Slower to heal due to moisture and bacteria in the mouth. Swelling of tongue common.
Cheek	Piercing in the cheek to simulate the look of a dimple. Requires internal and external care. Avoid facial hair removers during healing.
Labret	Piercing under the lower lip in the center. Requires external and internal care. Watch for tissue growth around the piercing.
Medusa	A mirror image of the labret with jewelry in the center dimple above the middle of the upper lip.

BODY PIERCINGS

Location of piercing	General information
Nasal septum	Piercing through the center of the nose in the soft tissue in front of the cartilage. Meticulous care required.
Jungle (Underside of nose)	Vertical piercing through the septum and out through the underside center of the nose. Requires pierced and stretched septum.
Nose	Any piercing of the soft tissue on the outside of the nose. Difficult healing due to bacteria in the nose.
Naval	Piercing of the outside skin of the belly button. Easier to pierce "innies," than "outies."
Nipples	Piercing inserted at the base of the nipple where it meets the areola.
Genitals	It is strongly recommended that you discuss any piercing with your gynecologist, urologist, and dermatologist.
Web space	Usually placed in the web space between the thumb and index finger. Special jewelry may be required.

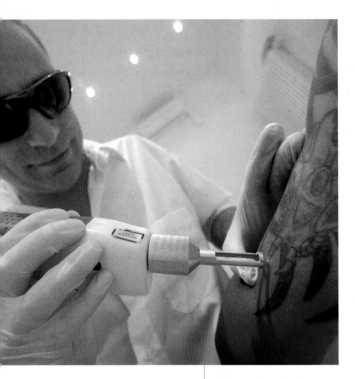

A variety of lasers are used to remove tattoo pigments.

Tattoos are now most commonly removed using lasers. The pigment in the tattoo serves as the target, or chromophore, for the laser in a process called selective photothermolysis. This means that the laser emits a specific wavelength of light that is absorbed by the tattoo pigment but not by the surrounding tissue. The pigment heats up and is destroyed while causing little damage to the surrounding skin. Scavenger cells in your body called macrophages come along and remove the pigment fragments.

Tattoos are usually made up of different ink colors. So, it is sometimes necessary to use more than one laser to remove one tattoo, depending on its design. The Q-switched ruby laser is used to remove blue and black tattoos pigments. The Q-switched alexandrite laser is also effective at removing black and blue pigments. In addition, it is able to remove green pigments. The Q-switched Nd:YAG can be used for blue, black and red pigments.

Laser treatments are not typically very painful. Many doctors will have you use a topical numbing cream prior to the treatment. In addition, many lasers make use of cooling systems to minimize the discomfort of the treatment. Several sessions will be required, there is discomfort during the process, and the cost may be prohibitive. Some dyes do not respond well to the laser, and scarring may occur. The size of the tattoo, the types of pigments and colors used, the depth of placement, and the amount of pigmentation in your skin all play a role in how successfully your tattoo will be removed. Patients are usually treated every six to eight weeks until the lesion is as clear as possible. While technology has come a long way, there is still no guarantee that any tattoo can be completely removed with a laser. Few doctors still cut out unwanted tattoos surgically or sand them off with dermabrasion. The bottom line is that you should be certain that you will still want the tattoo in 10 or 20 years and beyond. If you are not sure, don't get it done.

Hair removal

As you may remember from biology class, humans are mammals, and only mammals grow hair. Most people are happy about the hair that grows on top of the head. You may part it, braid it, curl it, pull it back, cut it short, wear it long or put bows in it. However, facial hair and body hair are another matter. Of course there are differences in the social norms for men and women.

While adolescent young men look forward to the day that they have enough facial hair to wear a full moustache or beard, most women are far less proud of the day that they have to tweeze their first hair on the upper lip or chin.

However, this facial hair is a reality for many women. Likewise, many men do seek to remove their facial hair and even some of their body hair, especially if they have a lot of it. More often than not, however, it is women who are most concerned with removing the hair of the eyebrows, under the arms, on the legs and in the bikini area. This section explores the different methods of hair removal.

Shaving

Shaving is one of the easiest, least expensive and least painful ways for men and women to remove hair anywhere on the body. A razor blade is guided along the surface of the skin to cut unwanted hair even with the skin's surface. It does not take long for the remaining hairs to grow above the surface of the skin. Even within a day or two these hairs are able to be seen and felt. The coarse, shaved hairs are commonly referred to as stubble when they first start to grow in.

Manual razor blades are used on moist skin. Ideally the skin is also treated with a shaving cream which helps to soften the hairs, protect the skin from the razor, and enable to razor to slide more effortlessly across the skin. Each razor may contain one or more blades, with some commercially available products now boasting up to four blades. Manual razors provide a close shave and smooth result, with multiple blades providing an even closer shave. Some people find that their skin is irritated by manual razors.

Electric razors are used on dry skin. Rotary razors have two or three blades that move in circles. Foil razors have blades that move from side to side. A protective mesh or "foil" covers the blade to protect the skin from the razor. Electric razors do not provide the same close shave that manual razors do, but they are also less irritating. Some men who are prone to razor bumps find that electric razors cause less of a problem for them than manual razors because the shave is not as close.

Aftershave may be used after either a wet shave or a dry shave. This product helps to

SKIN SOLUTION

Use a good shaving cream to get a smooth shave and minimize irritation. Look for one that makes an abundant lather and lubricates your skin well so that your razor glides easily over your skin.

Shaving is the easiest and cheapest way to remove unwanted hair. However, the effects only last a few days at best.

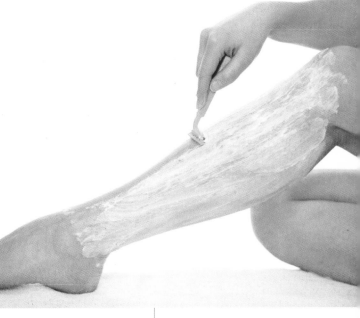

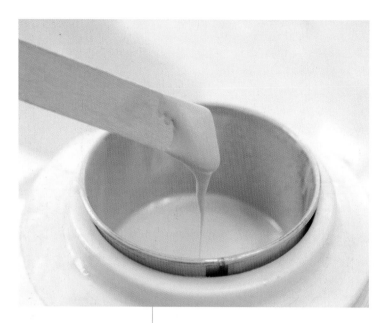

Hair removed by waxing takes several weeks to grow back.

close the pores. Aftershave often contains alcohol to minimize infection if the skin has any cuts, moisturizers to soften the skin, and fragrance.

Waxing

Waxing involves embedding unwanted hairs in wax, then removing the wax from the skin and taking the hairs with it in the process. Most products use beeswax or paraffin as the main ingredient. There are two types of waxing. In hot waxing, the product is melted and the hot wax is applied directly to the skin. A piece of fabric is placed over the wax. As the wax cools, it adheres to both the hairs and the fabric. The fabric is the pulled swiftly from the skin, taking the hardened wax and the hairs with it. In the cold waxing process, the wax product is already applied to fabric strips that are placed firmly on the skin. Similarly, the fabric strips are then removed from the skin taking the hairs with them. While the cold waxing is less painful than the hot wax, it is also less effective and generally requires more applications of the product.

Because waxing removes the entire length of the hair shaft, the results tend to last for a few weeks. It is an effective method both for small areas like the upper lip, and for larger areas like the underarms or the bikini area. Waxing can be painful, particularly hot waxing. People with sensitive skin may want to try cold waxing before attempting hot waxing. Also, people using irritating acne medications such as tretinoin or adapalene should discontinue their topical medications at least three or four days before a waxing treatment.

Threading

Threading is one of the oldest hair removal techniques and is practiced around the world. It involves using cotton thread to clip unwanted hair. A skilled practitioner holds a loop of thread which is twisted in the middle gently on the surface of the skin. The twists in the thread are moved back and forth along the length of the thread, cutting the hairs it comes in contact with along the way. This method is used primarily for facial hair but can also be used elsewhere on the body. Threading is particularly good for people who have sensitive skin or who are on acne treatment medications and have difficulty tolerating waxing.

Tweezing

Tweezers are used to pluck hairs from the root one-by-one. This is an effective method of hair removal for small areas such as the eyebrows, or for a few stray hairs on the upper lip, chin or neck. Because tweezing pulls the entire hair out, new hair takes longer to regrow when compared with shaving or threading. Hairs should be pulled in the direction in which they grow for the easiest removal.

Depilatories

Depilatories are chemicals that degrade the hair by causing swelling of the hair shaft and by breaking the disulfide bonds that provide its strength. These weakened hairs are then mechanically removed by wiping them off the skin. Similar to shaving, depilatories remove the hair at the level of the skin's surface so that the hairs do regrow fairly quickly. Unlike shaving which leaves the hairs with sharply cut ends, depilatories leave the hairs with blunted ends because of the degradation of the hair. These blunted hairs are less apt to cause razor bumps than the shaved hairs are.

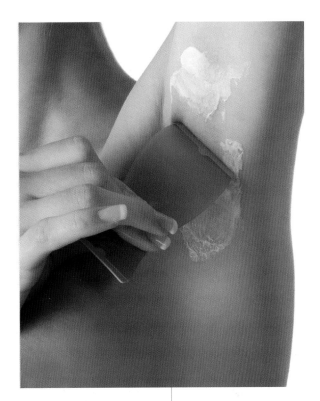

Some people find depilatories irritating to the skin. If you have this problem you can look for products specifically for sensitive skin.

Common active ingredients in depilatories include calcium thioglycolate, barium sulfide, sodium hydroxide, and potassium hydroxide. Depilatory products are available in many different forms, including creams, lotions, and powders. Depilatories may be used anywhere on the body. However, formulations for the face are generally milder than those for the body due to the sensitive nature of the facial skin. Because people commonly have irritation or allergy to these products, it is wise to perform a test before applying the product widely on the body. Place a small amount of product on the inner arm for five to ten minutes to see if any irritation or rash develops.

Shaving and depilatories remove the hair at skin level, not from the root, so you will start to see hair above the skin surface the next day, or in a few days at best.

Abrasives

Abrasives are only occasionally used for hair removal. Materials such as fine sandpaper, pumice stones, and aluminum oxide crystals are rubbed against

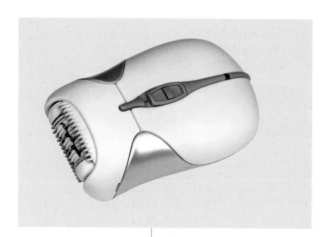

Epilators function like a row of tweezers that rotate and pull the hairs out by the root.

moist, soapy skin to break off the unwanted hairs. The abrasive surface is sometimes fashioned into a glove or a device for ease of use. This method is best used for areas such as the legs, which are less likely to develop irritation than sensitive areas like the face. Using abrasives may result in irritation of the underlying skin.

Epilators

An epilator is a device used to pull hairs out. Older models used rotating springs which would trap the hairs. Newer models trap the hairs between metal plates and pull them out, essentially functioning like electronic tweezers. Fans of these products note fewer ingrown hairs than with shaving. As with other methods of hair removal, these devices can be painful.

Electrolysis

Electrolysis is recognized as a method of permanent hair removal. In this process, a fine needle-like probe is inserted into the follicle of hairs in the anagen phase. Either direct current (DC) or alternating current (AC), or both are used in electrolysis processes termed galvonic electrolysis, thermolysis and blend. In either case, the current destroys the hair follicle such that it no longer grows hair. Galvonic electrolysis is more effective at destroying the follicle but is not as rapid as thermolysis. While electrolysis is an effective method of long-term hair removal it can be quite time–consuming since it treats just one hair follicle at a time.

Eflornithine cream

Eflornithine cream is available by prescription from a physician. It works to slow the growth of unwanted facial hair in women when applied twice a day. Some patients see results as early as one to two months into treatment, though for others it takes longer. You can usually tell how well the cream is working for you within six months of treatment. It is safe to use other forms of hair removal in conjunction with eflornithine cream. In fact, for the first few months it will be necessary to continue another form of hair removal until the cream reaches its maximum effect. Once the peak level of hair reduction is reached, some women only need the eflornithine cream. Others will still require some, although less frequent, other treatments.

Eflornithine is a prescription cream that slows down hair growth. You have to keep using it indefinitely in order to maintain your results.

Some patients notice stinging, burning, itching, dryness, irritation, or acne in the area where the cream is applied. If you experience these symptoms you should discuss it with your physician. Depending on the type and severity of the reaction he or she may suggest decreasing use to once a day. Or the medication may be discontinued altogether.

It is important to know that if you have a good result from eflornithine cream then you must continue to use it to maintain the results. If you stop using the cream the unwanted facial hair returns over time. However, you will not be hairier than you were before you started the cream.

Eflornithine cream is sometimes used by physicians to treat male patients. This is particularly true for men who get razor bumps. While this cream may not reduce hair growth as dramatically in men as it does in women, it often reduces the hair growth enough to provide improvement in the razor bumps.

Laser hair removal

Laser hair removal has become an incredibly popular procedure over the last ten years or so. Through advancements in laser technology and many years of research, this method has become a safe and effective method of long-term hair removal for many people.

Laser hair removal works by a process called selective photothermolysis. This means that the laser selectively targets melanin pigment, heats it and destroys it. Melanin is found both in the hair as well as in the region of the follicle responsible for new hair growth called the bulge. So, the laser's energy affects both the existing hair as well as the follicle's ability to produce new hairs.

There are actually two types of pigment in the hair. Eumelanin imparts brown and black color, while pheomelanin is responsible for blonde and red color. Lasers target the darker hues of the eumelanin, so it is more difficult to treat blonde hairs, red hairs and grey hairs with lasers than it is to treat darker hair. It is important to know that the same pigment that imparts color to hair also gives skin its color. The laser targets the pigment, not the hair itself. So if you have brown skin and brown hair, treatment must proceed cautiously with an experienced

SKIN SOLUTION

Laser hair removal works best for people who have dark hair and light skin. Lasers can cause discoloration on dark or tanned skin, so it is best to proceed with caution and make sure you visit an experienced professional.

Laser hair removal is usually performed monthly for four to eight sessions; you may require periodic touch-ups later.

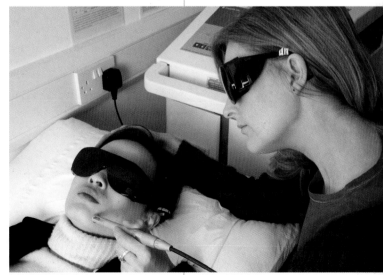

COMMON HAIR REMOVAL LASERS	
Laser	**Description**
Alexandrite	Very effective laser that is safest on light skin
Diode	Treats light to medium skin tones
Nd:YAG	Safest on all skin types

provider who has the right laser for your skin type.

There are several different types of lasers that are used for hair removal. It is important that you ask your treatment provider whether or not the type of laser they use is right for you. Specifically, you want to know if the laser is safe for your skin color and effective for your hair color and type.

Your provider may suggest doing a test spot before proceeding with treatment to see how your skin responds to the laser. Once treatment begins, you can expect to require several treatments to achieve initial clearing of the hair in the desired treatment area. The specific number of treatments varies, but most people can expect five to eight treatments to achieve the desired results. Each provider has his or her own protocol, but these treatments are usually spaced out by several weeks. There may also be medications that your provider prescribes before or after treatment. While the results of laser hair removal are long-term, they are not always permanent. It is common for people to require periodic touch-up treatments, sometimes even yearly.

No procedure is without its risks. Those associated with laser hair removal include scarring of the skin, dark or light discoloration of the skin, and bruising. These risks should be discussed with your provider prior to beginning treatment.

Makeup

You may wonder how to select the right makeup products. There are many factors that you should consider. Does a particular brand offer the shade selection that you are looking for? Does the product perform the way you want it to? Is it easy to apply? What price range does your budget allow? Does the makeup cause you any skin problems?

Ultimately there is not one "best" makeup. If you find a product that you like and that provides the desired effect, then it is a perfectly suitable product for you if it does not cause you any problems.

Caring for your makeup products

The first step in avoiding skin problems is taking good care of your makeup and applicators.

Makeup should always be stored covered with the lid or cap provided in a cool, dry place to minimize the growth of bacteria. Your products are not good indefinitely; use them only until they have reached their shelf life. You may want to use a permanent marker to note when you open a new product on the packaging so that you know when the product has become too old to use. The guidelines here are approximate. If you notice that a product has developed an odor or has changed color or consistency before its shelf life has expired then it is time to throw that product away.

Makeup brushes should be washed every two to four weeks. You can use your regular shampoo, or purchase shampoo that is specially formulated to be gentle for your makeup brushes. Wet the brush with warm water, then use a small amount of shampoo to generate a lather. If you wash your brushes at night, you can let them air dry and they will be ready to go for you the next morning.

If you prefer to use a sponge to apply liquid or cream makeup or even powder, you may consider buying inexpensive disposable sponges that can be discarded every few days. Sponges store moisture and are a breeding ground for bacteria. If you reuse sponges more than two or three days in a row you should wash the sponge with soap and water and allow it to air dry.

Taking it off

Your makeup is formulated to stay in place for long periods of time in order to minimize your need to re-apply during the course of the day. However, when bedtime approaches you want to make sure that you remove all of your makeup. Leaving it on can cause acne breakouts. The challenge in removing the makeup is that mild facial cleansers are often not strong enough to thoroughly wash off all cosmetic products. Waterproof eye makeup such as eyeliner and mascara can be particularly difficult to remove, and the eyelid skin is delicate skin and less tolerant of prolonged scrubbing. Foundations and face powders can also

SHELF LIFE OF MAKEUP PRODUCTS	
Liquid eye makeup: mascara, eyeliner	3 months
Liquids: foundation, concealer	1 years
Nail polish	1 year
Creams: eye shadow, blush, foundation	1.5 years
Lipstick and lip gloss	2 years
Pencils: eye, lip	2 years
Powders: eye, cheek, bronzer	2 years

A variety of brushes are available to help you apply your makeup; they are made with natural or synthetic fibers.

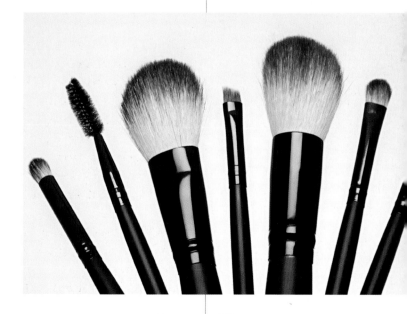

require special attention to remove well. Makeup remover is an essential product for people who wear color cosmetics. It whisks away the otherwise hard to remove products. Makeup remover is usually found as a liquid that you can apply with a cotton ball or cotton square. Some companies make presoaked wipes that are particularly handy for travel or to keep in your purse for unexpected late nights. Some products are formulated specifically for eye makeup removal. Others are for all makeup. Select a product depending on which cosmetics you use. After using a full face product you can splash your face with water or follow up with a mild cleanser.

Presoaked makeup remover wipes gently remove cosmetics, dirt, and oil from the face, and are especially handy when you are traveling.

Avoiding makeup mishaps

If you find that repeated use of a makeup product causes redness, itching, or rash, you may be allergic to that product. If you believe that you are allergic to a product or an ingredient, you should see your dermatologist who may opt to perform a patch test to investigate your reaction. Sometimes specific ingredients are able to be identified. Fragrance and preservatives are common allergens found in makeup products. Knowing what you are allergic to will help you to read labels before making a new purchase. If you are not aware of a specific ingredient that you are allergic to, you should look for products labeled "hypoallergenic."

Some makeup products can clog the pores and cause blackheads or whiteheads, also known as comedones. This is particularly true of foundations. If you are acne-prone, or if the makeup you are using is causing pimples, then you should look for products that are noncomedogenic.

This means that it doesn't cause blackheads and whiteheads. Looking for products that are oil-free will also help keep you from developing blemishes. Eye makeup should never, ever be shared. This is especially important with mascara wands and eyeliner pencils, both of which come in contact with the moist surface of the eye. Bacteria

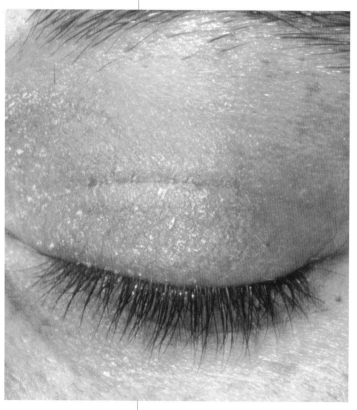

Eyelid skin is particularly delicate and is prone to irritation from cosmetic products.

and viruses are easily spread from one person's eye to another. The result is an infection of the eye called conjunctivitis, commonly called "pink eye."

Permanent makeup

Have you lost your eyebrows and lashes due to alopecia areata or chemotherapy? Or maybe you have a scar that you would like to conceal? Or perhaps you are just tired of applying your makeup every single day? If the answer to any of these questions is yes, then permanent makeup might be a good option for you.

Permanent makeup uses tattoo pigments placed into the dermis to provide the appearance of wearing makeup. These tattoos can mimic eyeliner, eyebrows, lip liner, lip color or camouflage scars and discoloration. However, unlike cosmetic products that you can wash off and re-apply if you are not happy with their appearance, these tattoos are for keeps. So, it is very important that you choose an experienced person to apply the permanent makeup. Ask to see before and after photos of other clients, and to provide references.

When permanent makeup is first applied it can look a bit exaggerated. Over time the pigment settles and the look becomes less harsh and obvious. For some people the pigments will really start to fade over time, requiring touch-up treatments years down the road.

It is important to know that there are certain risks involved with the use of permanent makeup. Some people are allergic to the pigments. Others develop keloids in the location of the injection. And infections can be spread if the technician does not maintain and sterilize the equipment properly. In order to minimize bad outcomes, you should have a thorough consultation with your technician prior to beginning application of the permanent makeup.

SKIN SOLUTION
If you have sensitive skin, look for cosmetic products that are hypoallergenic, noncomedogenic, and fragrance free to minimize the chances that you will have a reaction.

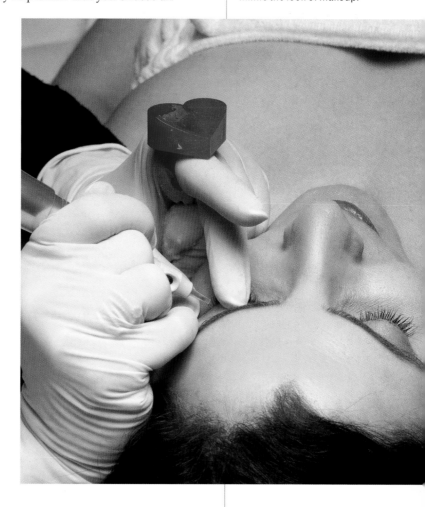

Strategically placed tattoo pigments can mimic the look of makeup.

Common Skin Diseases: From A to Z

3

There are a number of skin conditions that you will encounter over your lifetime. This chapter explores the most common skin diseases and presents an overview of treatment options. There are over two thousand diseases that can affect the skin, so this is not a substitute for a visit to your dermatologist. Any new or persistent skin condition should be evaluated by a professional.

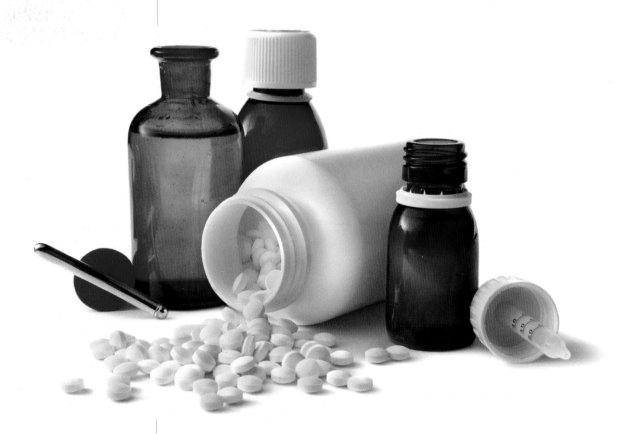

Acanthosis nigricans

You have probably seen this common skin problem, even if you have never heard of it. The velvety brown discoloration that appears on the back of the neck, under the arms, or in the groin cannot simply be washed off, because it's not dirt. Acanthosis nigricans is most commonly found in people who are overweight or who have diabetes; conditions in which the level of insulin are elevated. Often the body does not respond properly to insulin, a condition that is called insulin resistance. The skin cells are stimulated by the elevated insulin level, to produce the dark thickened patches.

Before you get treatment for acanthosis nigricans, it is important to have your doctor check your blood for insulin resistance and diabetes. If you show signs of these disorders, the appropriate medication can be given. If you are above your ideal weight, think of this as a sign to begin watching what you eat, and exercising to improve your health and skin.

Acanthosis nigricans can be treated with various topical creams and lotions. These include prescription tretinoin cream, hydroquinone cream, and topical steroids, alone or in combination. It is sometimes improved by over-the-counter lotions containing urea, alpha hydroxy acids, lactic acid, or salicylic acid.

Acne

Who hasn't had a pimple or two at one time or another? Acne is one of the most common skin diseases. It can start in the pre-teen years, during adolescence, or in early adulthood. For some people it lasts a few years while for others it can last for a decade or two, persisting into the forties and beyond. Did you know there are different types of pimples, and one person may get any or all of them? Open and closed comedones, inflammatory papules, pustules, and cystic nodules are all common types of pimples. Open comedones are commonly referred to as blackheads, and closed comedones are also called whiteheads. These pimples have a visible plug of debris that you may be tempted to squeeze out, but you should resist this urge. Inflammatory papules are the pink pimples, which may be tender to the touch. You may get pus-filled pimples, which are called pustules, and also should not be picked or squeezed. Cystic nodules are the painful bumps that lie below the surface of the skin. Any of these lesions can occur on the face chest, shoulders, or back.

Acne can be caused by a combination of factors. The three main factors are bacteria on the skin, the amount of oil the skin produces, and how easily

---

Skin Myth

True or False?
The severity and duration of acne are the same for both men and women.

False

In fact, young teenage men tend to have worse acne than young teenage women. However, acne is more likely to persist into the thirties and even the forties for women.

OVER-THE-COUNTER ACNE TREATMENTS

There are a wide range of products available without a prescription to treat your acne. Ingredients to look for include:

- **Benzoyl peroxide**
- **Nicotinamide gel**
- **Resorcinol**
- **Salicylic acid**
- **Sulfur**
- **Triclosan**
- **Tea tree oil**

the pores are clogged. Each of us has bacteria on the skin. This is normal and does not mean that your skin is dirty. These bacteria "feed" on the oil produced by the skin and release factors that cause inflammation. In addition, people who are acne-prone have skin cells that tend to be sticky and block the pores.

Many over-the-counter products are effective in treating mild acne. Ingredients to look for include benzoyl peroxide 2.5 to 10 percent, salicylic acid 2 percent, sulfur 5 to 8 percent and resorcinol 2 percent. Tea tree oil is a natural ingredient that can also be used to control mild outbreaks. These active ingredients can be found in a wide variety of products including face washes, toners, masques, and leave-on creams and gels.

Acne treatments often leave the skin feeling dry. This can be minimized by using the medication every other day for two weeks to give your skin a chance to acclimate to the medicine. Then, you can increase to daily use.

Acne treatments should be applied to a clean face both in the morning and at night. So, it's important to wash your face twice a day, if you are acne-prone. This is especially true if you wear makeup. Liquid makeup removers

SKIN SOLUTION

A noncomedogenic moisturizer can be used on your face after acne treatment is applied if you find that the medication is too drying to the skin. Noncomedogenic is a term applied to makeup and skin-care products that do not block pores.

It is important to wash your face twice daily to ensure that you keep your acne-prone skin free of dirt and oil.

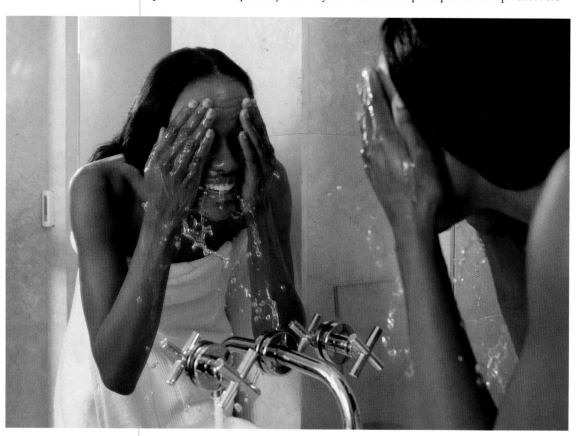

can be used on a tissue or cotton ball, and presoaked wipes are also available. It is important to look for products that are marked noncomedogenic.

If over-the-counter medications have proven ineffective for you, there are several prescription products also available. Retinoids are derived from vitamin A and are particularly good at unclogging pores. Topical retinoids include tretinoin, adapelene, and tazarotene. Topical or oral antibiotics may also be used to control acne. These include topical clindamycin and erythromycin, and oral tetracycline, minocycline and doxycycline. Other oral antibiotics are often used for patients who are allergic to tetracyclines or who have not had a satisfactory response to them. Other topical prescription medications include azeleic acid, salicylic acid 6 percent and topical dapsone. If your doctor believes that your hormones are a cause of acne, she may prescribe oral contraceptives or other hormonal treatments such as spironolactone.

Some physicians treat acne with a laserlike device called the IPL. Others may suggest chemical peels with agents such as salicylic acid, glycolic acid, lactic acid, or thricholoacetic acid (TCA). TCA peels should be used with caution in patients with richly pigmented skin. The chemical peels are useful not only for controlling the acne but also for helping to fade the pink spots that are left behind in Caucasian skin and the dark spots that are common in brown skin.

The most severe or recalcitrant cases of acne may be treated with a medication called isotretinoin. This medication is very effective, but it can have serious side effects. Careful screening is needed to identify appropriate patients, and monthly monitoring is required. Monitoring includes a visit to your physician for a physical examination to evaluate your progress on the medication, and discussion to evaluate side effects and psychological well-being. A monthly pregnancy test is necessary for women, and your doctor may order

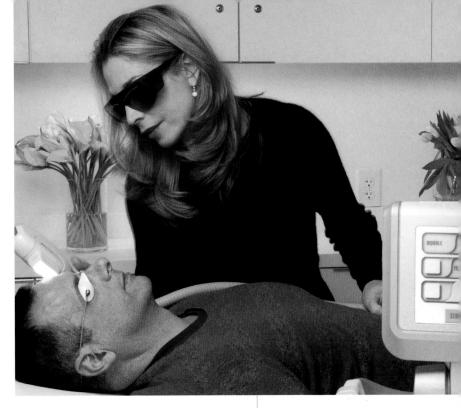

A patient undergoing IPL (intense pulsed light) treatment for treatment of his acne.

Use a makeup remover to thoroughly remove cosmetics from your face before bedtime in order to help prevent blemishes.

other blood work to check on your liver enzymes and your triglycerides. Isotretinoin is not appropriate for pregnant women because its effects on an unborn child are severe.

Acne is very common during pregnancy because of the hormonal changes associated with it. Some women who have never had acne before develop it for the first time. There are only a few acne medicines that can be used safely during pregnancy. These include topical erythromycin and azeleic acid. Products containing glycolic acid can be used to unclog the pores. Your obstetrician/gynecologist should be made aware of any medications you are using.

Actinic keratosis

Have you spent too much time in the sun without adequate protection? One of the most common forms of sun damage is a small growth called an actinic keratosis (AK). These spots are important because they are precancerous, each with a chance of turning into a squamous cell skin cancer. Because of this risk, all AKs should be treated by a doctor.

Actinic keratoses are sometimes easier to feel than they are to see.

AKs are characterized by a slightly rough patch of skin that may appear pink, red, or flesh-colored. They are usually between 1 and 5 millimeters in size but are sometimers larger. Often people first notice a patch of rough, dry skin that does not seem to go away despite the application of moisturizer. Some people have just one; others have several AKs at a time.

Most dermatologists can diagnose AKs by sight and feel. Occasionally a biopsy will be necessary to make sure that the spot has not already become cancerous. AKs may be frozen off using liquid nitrogen cryotherapy. If you have several lesions, you may be prescribed a topical prescription medication such as 5-fluorouracil cream, immiquimod cream, or diclofenac sodium gel. Occasionally extensive AKs are treated with chemical peels or lasers.

Skin Myth

True or False?
Actinic keratoses are rough, dry spots that can be treated with moisturizers.

False

In fact, AKs feel rough and dry but do not go away with moisturizers. They need to be treated by a doctor with liquid nitrogen spray or prescription cream because they can turn into squamous cell skin cancers.

Blisters

Blisters are a common problem that can occur as the result of many different skin conditions. Almost everyone has had a blister on the foot from wearing a new pair of shoes. This type of blister, which occurs from the rubbing of the shoe against the foot, is called a friction blister and is the most common of these uncomfortable lesions.

While most blisters are harmless, those that are surrounded by skin that is red, swollen, and warm to the touch may be the result of a bacterial infection, in which case prescription antibiotics are needed. If you repeatedly develop unexplainable blisters on different parts of the body, then you should see a doctor. There are uncommon but serious diseases such as pemphigus vulgaris and bullous pemphigoid that your doctor will need to test you for.

If you want to pop your blister, you can use a clean pin to make a small hole in the roof of the blister to let the fluid out. Try to leave the roof of the blister intact to protect the skin underneath from becoming infected.

CAUSES OF BLISTERS
Friction
Burns
Dermatitis
Bug bites
Bacterial or viral infection
Blistering diseases

Bug bites

The itchy nuisance of bug bites is something you have probably experienced countless times. As with many other conditions, prevention is best. If you are going to be outdoors, particularly in wooded areas, wear long sleeves and long pants. Use an insect repellent on any areas where your skin is exposed. The Centers for Disease Control (CDC) recommends using products containing DEET or picaridin.

If this advice comes too late and you have already served as a meal for a little creature, try over-the-counter antihistamines such as diphenhydramine, loratadine, or cetirizine to reduce the itch. Acetaminophen or ibuprofen can be used to reduce pain. Topical hydrocortisone cream can be used to reduce inflammation, and antibacterial ointments can be used over any open areas to minimize the risk of infection. If this does not provide sufficient relief, then you should see your doctor for prescription medications.

COMMON INSECT BITES	
Insect	**Usual bite appearance**
Mosquito	One or more red hivelike lesions
Bed bugs	Bites occur in clusters of three
Fire ants	Painful pustules and hivelike lesions
Fleas	Hivelike spots with a central punctum
Ticks	Engorged tick may be visible on the skin; bulls-eye, targetoid rash called erythema chronicum migrans may be present if the infectious Lyme disease is transmitted.
Black widow spider	Two fang marks are visible
Brown recluse spider	Red, white, and blue sign: blue-black necrotic center surrounded by a pale ring and an outermost circle of redness

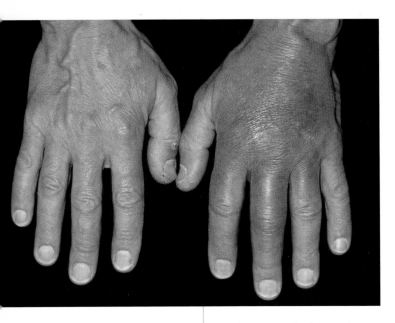

Cellulitis

Cellulitis is a deep infection of the skin, involving the dermis and the soft tissue below the skin. If you have a localized rash displaying the common signs of redness, swelling, warmth to touch, and pain, then you may have cellulitis. You may not feel well in general, and you may even have a fever or chills.

These infections occur most commonly on the leg in adults and on the face in children. Cellulitis may spread rapidly and requires immediate attention. Antibiotics are used to treat cellulitis. Oral antibiotics are often sufficient, but some people will require intravenous antibiotics in the hospital.

Staphylococci and streptococci are the organisms that are the most common cause of these infections. The bacteria can enter through any break in the skin, including cuts, insect bites, skin compromised by eczema or athlete's foot, surgical sites, or intravenous injection sites. Diabetics, people with chronic leg swelling, IV drug users, and people whose immune systems are compromised are at increased risk for developing cellulitis.

Cellulitis occurs most commonly on the leg but can affect other areas of the body as well.

Dermatosis papulosa nigra

Dermatosis papulosa nigra (DPNs) are brown growths that appear to sit on the surface of the skin and multiply with each passing year. Sometimes called "flesh moles," they occur most often on the face and neck of individuals with tan or brown skin tones. These lesions have absolutely no cancerous potential. They are usually small, about the size of the head of a pin, but can enlarge to the size of a dime. Some people don't like the way their DPNs look and opt for elective, cosmetic treatment to remove them. This procedure can be performed easily by your dermatologist or plastic surgeon. There are three common methods of removal: snipping with surgical scissors, "burning" with the electric needle, or freezing with liquid nitrogen. Freezing DPNs with liquid nitrogen is an acceptable treatment for lighter skin tones, but it is not appropriate for darker skin because it can lead to

Dermatosis papulosa nigra lesions are not contagious, which means that you cannot spread them by touching them. DPNs run in families and can be inherited.

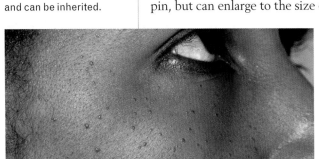

discolorations. All methods of removal cause some minimal discomfort, but a topical numbing medication can be used to make the procedure painless. New DPNs will develop over time, so be prepared to visit your dermatologist every year or two for a touch-up removal.

Eczema

Eczema is a very common condition that causes itchy skin and a red rash. It is also called dermatitis, which simply means inflammation of the skin. Many people develop eczema in infancy. About half of the people who develop eczema as a baby will grow out of it. Other people may develop eczema later in life. There is no cure for eczema, but it can usually be controlled quite effectively. The rash may come and go, and for most sufferers, eczema is worse in the winter.

Eczema can occur anywhere on the body. Usual areas include flexures, which are areas where the skin folds in, notably the neck, the bend of the arm, and behind the knee. Facial, hand, or foot eczema often occur in children.

Generally people who have eczema have dry skin. So taking good care of the skin is an important step toward minimizing flare-ups. People with eczema should take lukewarm baths or showers and should stay in the water for only 5 to 10 minutes. Long, hot soaks may be good for the soul, but they are bad for the skin. In addition, your choice of cleanser is very important. Look for moisturizing body washes or synthetic detergent bars to keep your skin from drying out.

TYPES OF ECZEMA	TREATMENT
Atopic dermatitis	Begins in infancy; half of children will outgrow it.
Contact dermatitis	Results from coming into contact with something you are allergic to such as nickel, or something that irritated the skin, like hand soap that is not properly rinsed from under a ring.
Dyshydrotic eczema	Small water blisters are seen on the palms of the hands or the soles of the feet.
Nummular dermatitis	Round, itchy patches can appear anywhere on the body.
Stasis dermatitis	Legs that are chronically swollen develop an overlying itchy rash.

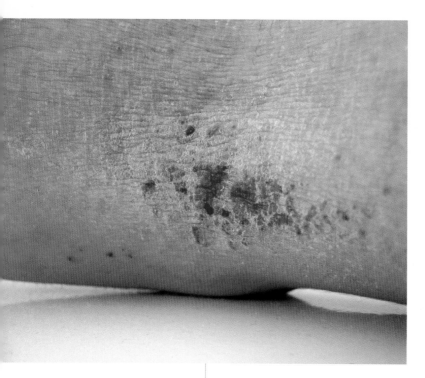

If an itchy rash persists for more than a week and is not controlled by over-the-counter hydrocortisone 1 percent cream or ointment, it is time to see a physician. Your dermatologist may prescribe topical steroids in the form of cream, ointment, solution, gel, or foam preparation. Or he or she may prescribe a steroid sparing agent such as tacrolimus or pemicrolimus. Severe cases may be treated with narrow-band UVB light treatment or with prednisone or other oral immune suppressants.

People with eczema are very itchy. Over-the-counter medicines such as diphenhydramine (Benadryl) may be effective in controlling itch, or your physician may prescribe itch pills such as hydroxyzine or other antihistamines to keep you comfortable. You should be careful, however, because many itch pills can make you drowsy. Start by taking them in the evening to see how they affect you and do not drive a car or operate heavy machinery until you are sure that you are not drowsy.

Eczema is not contagious, but people who suffer from it are more prone to developing bacterial or viral infections of the skin when their disease is active.

Epidermoid cyst

These firm, round growths are located below the surface of the skin in the dermis. This means that you may be able to feel an epidermoid cyst before you can see it. They may range from just a few millimeters to several centimeters in size. Sometimes the skin over the cyst is smooth, but there may be a central pore visible. They can occur anywhere on the body, including the scalp, face, trunk, genital region, or on the extremities. Because these growths are harmless, they do not have to be treated, though they are easily excised.

Epidermoid cysts can become infected, in which case the overlying skin becomes pink or red, and the cyst may become tender. An infected cyst may be treated with oral antibiotics or with an incision and drainage. Cysts may become inflamed, in which case they are treated with an injection of steroids. The most definitive treatment involves cutting out the cyst under local anesthesia.

SKIN SOLUTION

Epidermoid cysts sometimes drain a foul-smelling substance with the consistency of cottage cheese. This is normal. If the skin around the cyst is red, warm to the touch, or painful, the cyst may be infected or may have ruptured beneath the surface of the skin. In this case, you should seek medical treatment.

TYPES OF FOLLICULITIS	
Bacterial folliculitis	Usually caused by Staphylococcus or Streptococcus
Hot tub folliculitis	Caused by the bacteria Pseudomonas which is found in hot tubs
Gram negative folliculitis	A form of bacteria seen in acne patients after prolonged treatment; caused by Klebsiella, Enterobacter, or Proteus
Pityrosporum folliculitis	This yeast most commonly causes folliculitis in young adults
Dermatophyte folliculitis	Usually caused by Trichophyton species, can be seen in the beard area of men or on the legs of women who shave
Demodex folliculitis	Caused by mites that live in the hair follicles
Herpes folliculitis	Usually seen in men who have a cold sore and spread the herpes virus to the hair follicles while shaving
Eosinophilic folliculitis	Seen in people who are HIV positive, this condition does not have an infectious organism associated with it

Folliculitis

Folliculitis is an infection of the hair follicles. It may be superficial, in which case you will probably see pink or red bumps, or pustules. This eruption may be itchy. Or, the infection may be deeper down in the follicle in which case you may see deep, painful boils that may be filled with pus. Folliculitis occurs when the follicles have been irritated, making them more prone to infection. Common causes of irritation to the follicles include friction from clothing, use of adhesive tape, or from exposure to irritating substances, such as sweat or makeup. Treatment for this condition depends on the organism that is causing the infection. Topical or oral antibiotics are used for bacterial infections. Antivirals, antifungals, or other treatments might be prescribed by your doctor depending on her suspicion regarding the causative organism.

Antibacterial soaps and over-the-counter acne washes may be useful in preventing flare-ups of folliculitis.

Fungal infections

Fungus really is among us. It is everywhere. While there are several different types of fungus that can cause skin infections, the two most common causes are discussed here. Candida is a yeast that causes a pink rash, often with "satellite" pustules noted just outside the boundaries of the rash. It is commonly seen in the skin folds, in the diaper area of young children, and in immunocompromised people. Candida can also be found in the mouth.

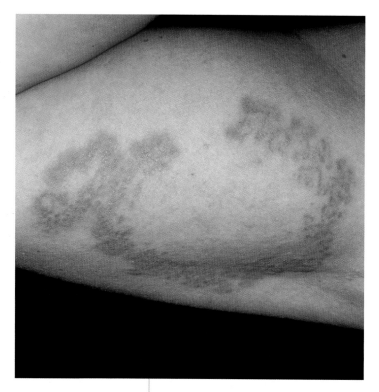

Dermatophytes are fungi that infect the superficial layers of the skin. These infections can occur anywhere on the body and are often itchy.

Depending on the location of the fungal infection, the suspected organism, and the amount of body surface area involved, your doctor might prescribe oral or topical antifungal medications.

Granuloma annulare

Granuloma annulare (GA) is a harmless rash that usually occurs in otherwise healthy people. The rash may be localized to one area of the body, or it may be generalized and involve a large portion of the skin's surface. The characteristic rash is composed of pink rings of individual tiny papules. In fact, it is sometimes mistaken for the fungal infection commonly referred to as ringworm. GA usually goes away on its own after a year or two. Localized lesions might be treated with topical steroids, or steroids injected into the spots. Widespread lesions are most commonly treated with topical steroids, oral retinoids, or light treatments. There are several second-line treatments that your doctor might try if you don't respond to one of these treatments.

Fungal infections are also called ringworm because they often have a ring-shaped appearance with raised edges, or a central clearing.

DERMATOPHYTE INFECTIONS

Name	Location	Common name
Tinea capitis	Scalp	Ringworm
Tinea corporis	Body	Ringworm
Tinea barbae	Beard	Barber's itch
Tinea cruris	Groin	Jock itch
Tinea pedis	Feet	Athlete's foot
Onychomycosis	Nails	Nail fungus

Herpes

Do you know that most people in the United States are infected with a herpes virus? Human herpes virus (HHV) type 1 is the most common cause of cold sores around the mouth. HHV type 2 is the most common cause of genital herpes. But some people have HHV 1 in the genital area and HHV 2 in the mouth. This distinction really doesn't matter since the problem that each virus causes in each area is similar.

Herpes eruptions begin as small water blisters called vesicles. These rupture fairly quickly and leave very superficial open wounds called erosions. Eventually these spots crust over and heal without leaving a scar. The vesicles and erosions are typically very painful. The first episode, or primary outbreak, is usually the worst, with the largest number of vesicles and the most discomfort.

Once a person has become infected with the herpes virus, there is no way to get rid of it. At first, recurrences usually happen frequently, but they tend to become less frequent over time. Stress tends to cause herpes to flare. Herpes is very contagious. It is transmitted by skin-to-skin contact. This can come from a kiss, from sexual intercourse, or from any contact with an infected area. For instance, dentists and dental hygienists who don't wear gloves may get herpes from their patients' mouths. This eruption of the finger is called herpetic whitlow. Newborns may become infected during delivery if the mother is infected. Neonatal herpes can be dangerous to a baby and is most likely to occur if a mother is experiencing a primary outbreak. Obstetricians will usually elect to perform a cesarean section to minimize the risk if a mother is having a herpes outbreak during delivery.

If you or your sexual partner has herpes, you should abstain from intercourse during times when there are active lesions to avoid spreading the disease. Even if there are no active legions, condoms should still be used during intercourse because the virus can still be spread.

There are good antiviral medications that can shorten the course of a herpes outbreak. Acyclovir, famcyclovir, and valacyclovir are all available by prescription. For people who get recurrences six times or more per year, suppressive therapy might be suggested. You can take a pill every day to avoid the recurrence.

Hives

Hives are raised, pink, itchy areas on the skin that may be just a few millimeters or several centimeters in size. They are also called wheals, and the medical name for the condition is urticaria. The most striking thing about hives, besides how much they itch, is the fact that each individual spot comes and goes very quickly, characteristically within 24 hours. People usually have several hives at one time, and new lesions

Skin Myth

True or False?
You can get herpes from a toilet seat.
False
In fact, the herpes virus does not survive on toilet seats and is transmitted only by skin-to-skin contact.

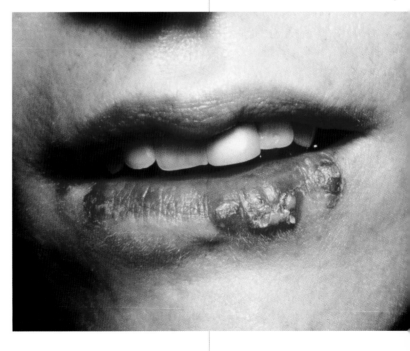

This painful cold sore caused by herpes simplex virus can sometimes be prevented by taking an antiviral medication at the first feeling of discomfort, which is called the prodrome.

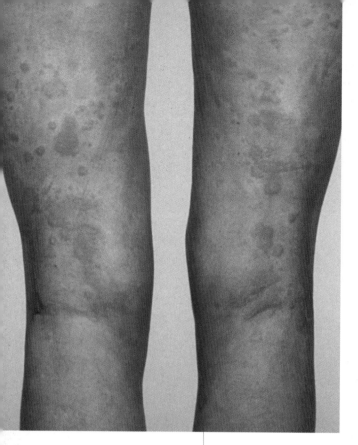

may continue to develop over long periods of time. Each spot represents a localized area of swelling in the dermis.

If you had hives for less than six weeks, you are considered to have "acute urticaria." If your hives have persisted continuously for more than six weeks, then you have "chronic urticaria." Causes of acute urticaria include a recent illness, such as an upper respiratory tract infection, or exposure to a medication or a certain trigger such as food. Chronic urticaria is often seen in response to a physical condition like heat, cold, stress, exercise, sun, water, pressure, or vibration. It may also be seen in association with autoimmune diseases such as thyroid disease, rheumatoid arthritis, or vitiligo. It is often difficult to pinpoint the reason why someone develops hives. If this is the case, then the condition is called "idiopathic." There are other serious problems that can mimic hives, including diseases that cause the skin to blister or cause problems with the blood vessels, so hives lasting more than a few days should be evaluated by a physician.

Individual hives come and go quickly, usually within 24 hours, but you may continue to develop new hives for days, weeks, months, or rarely even years.

Hives are most effectively treated by avoiding a trigger if one is identified. So if you know that tomatoes give you hives, for example, then don't eat tomatoes. Antihistamines are the mainstay of treatment for urticaria. Over-the-counter medications like diphenhydramine, ceterizine, and loratadine, available at your local pharmacy, can be quite helpful in controlling hives. They should be used according to the directions on the packaging. Prescription antihistamines, higher doses of antihistamines, or a combination of medications are sometimes needed and require a doctor's evaluation and prescription. If you have hives lasting more than a week or two, or hives that are not adequately controlled by over-the-counter medications, you should see your doctor.

SKIN SOLUTION
Use oatmeal from your pantry in your bath to soothe your itching hives. Aloe vera gel can also help relieve your symptoms.

Angioedema

Angioedema is a condition that is sometimes seen in people who get hives but may also occur without the presence of hives. While hives represent swelling of the dermis, angioedema is swelling of the deeper tissue. This is a potentially life-threatening condition that occurs in the face, neck, and genitals. Angioedema of the head and neck can include swelling of the lips, tongue, throat, eyelids, whole face, or any combination of these. Throat swelling can make it difficult to breathe, so if you develop angioedema, you should go to the nearest emergency room right away. People with a history of angioedema should carry epinephrine with them at all times. This medication is available by prescription from your physician.

Impetigo

Impetigo is a very common skin infection usually seen in children. It can also occur in adults who come into contact with infected children. The skin develops an infection with bacteria, usually of staphylococcus aureus or streptococcus pyogenes. While normal skin does a good job of resisting bacterial infection, skin that has been broken or has an active disease is more easily infected. So impetigo is often seen in children who have eczema, insect bites, varicella, or other skin diseases.

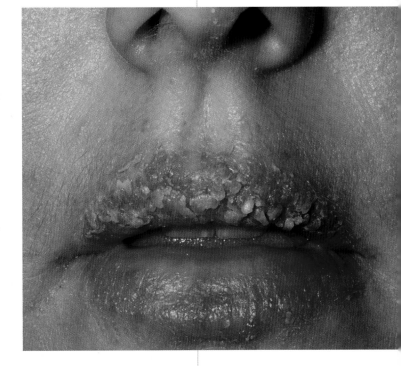

Impetigo can be recognized by its characteristic honey-colored yellow crust that forms over compromised areas of skin. Small or large blisters may also be present. Because impetigo is highly contagious, it should be treated right away. Physicians usually prescribe either antibacterial washes, topical antibiotic ointments, or oral antibiotics. People who get recurrent impetigo infections are sometimes carriers of staphylococcus aureus. Your doctor can check for this by doing a test that involves swabbing the inside of your nose to culture for bacteria. Carriers are usually treated with topical antibiotic ointments for several days.

Impetigo is found most commonly around the nose and mouth and is easily recognized by its honey-colored crust.

Intertrigo

Intertrigo refers to an inflammation of the skin folds, caused by the skin rubbing together. It is commonly seen under the breasts, under the arms, in the folds of the abdomen, and in the groin. It is most common in people who are overweight and in people with diabetes. The skin may be pink or red and may be slightly moist or even ooze clear fluid. The condition is aggravated by heat and may include symptoms of itching, stinging, or burning. Irritated skin makes a secondary infection more likely, so infections of candida, fungus, bacteria, or viruses may occur in areas of intertrigo.

Prevention is the best medicine, and intertrigo can usually be minimized by losing weight if you are overweight. Keeping the skin cool and dry by wearing natural fabrics such as cotton can be helpful. Using baby powder to absorb moisture and reduce friction can also minimize intertrigo flares. Skin protectants such as petrolatum (Vaseline) or zinc oxide can be helpful if the skin has started to break down. These are ingredients found in most diaper creams. Over-the-counter hydrocortisone cream may be useful in reducing inflammation and over-the-counter antifungal creams may minimize any fungal infection. If you are not able to control intertrigo with these treatments, you should see your dermatologist as prescription-strength treatments may be necessary.

Diaper rash creams form a protective barrier on the skin and can be used to control intertrigo.

Keloids

Scar tissue is formed as the skin repairs itself after it has been injured. Sometimes the scar tissue grows to extend beyond the size and boundaries of the original cut. This is called a keloid. Keloids are harmless growths that can be flesh colored, pink, purple, or brown. They can appear when the skin has been cut, for instance after a surgery, or after getting your ears pierced. They can also appear after the skin has been inflamed by conditions such as acne or razor bumps. Some people develop keloids spontaneously, without any preceding trauma to the skin. These spontaneous keloids often occur on the chest or back. Keloids appear more commonly in women than in men. That is largely because women get more ear piercings and other body piercings than men do. Keloids also occur more commonly in people with richly pigmented skin, although they can appear in people of any race or ethnicity. They tend to occur less frequently in children and in older adults.

Your keloids may not bother you at all. Sometimes they are itchy, and some people find them to be painful. Depending on the size and location of the keloid, they are often treatable. Treatment options should be discussed with your doctor.

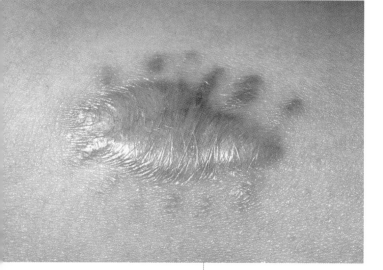

Treatment of keloids includes flattening the scar and reducing itching and pain.

TREATMENT OPTIONS FOR KELOIDS	
Treatment	**Comments**
Steroid injections	Best for small and medium-sized keloids
Surgical excision	Should be followed by steroid injections or radiation treatment to prevent recurrence
Cryotherapy	Freezing the skin using very cold liquid nitrogen is an effective treatment but may cause discoloration in pigmented skin
Laser	Pulsed dye laser or other lasers may be used to treat keloids, but treatment may be expensive
Silicone gel sheets	Covering keloids with these sheets can help to reduce the size of the keloid over time
Compression	Applying pressure to areas of keloid excision or to keloid-prone areas such as ear lobes that have just been pierced can help to prevent keloid formation
Medications	Your physician may try interferon, imiquimod, 5 flourouracil or bleomycin alone or in combination with other medications

Keratosis pilaris

Keratosis pilaris appears on the outside of the arms and on the thighs, buttocks, or back as small rough bumps. These bumps are similar to goose bumps, but unlike goose bumps they do not go away. The bumps may vary in color, and in some people they are skin-colored and in others they are red. Keratosis pilaris is caused by a thickening of the skin around the hair follicle.

The bumps of keratosis pilaris are stubborn to treat and often return after treatment.

Keratosis pilaris is one of the skin concerns that many people think will be improved by rubbing and scrubbing the skin. But vigorous washing will only irritate it. Since this is not a serious condition, treatment is not necessary; and some physicians think that it improves with age. However, most people do not like the appearance or feel of the skin. Although there is no cure for keratosis pilaris, there are several treatments that can help restore the smooth feel to the skin. Lotions and creams with ingredients that exfoliate the skin have been helpful

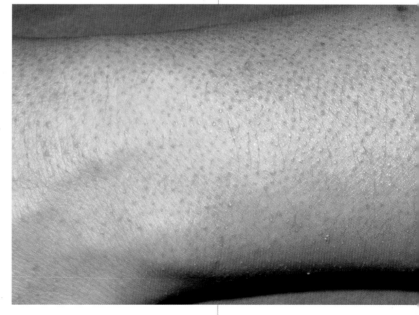

in smoothing the roughened skin of keratosis pilaris. Glycolic acid, lactic acid, salicylic acid, and urea have been found to be effective after several weeks of daily or twice-daily application. These creams and lotions should be used with caution, as they could lead to redness or irritation. Apply to completely dry skin and begin using only once a day so that your skin can adjust to them. Additionally, tretinoin can improve keratosis pilaris, but it should be used only once a day or every other day to prevent possible irritation.

Lice

There are three types of lice that can cause infestations in people. Pediculosis hominis var. capitis causes head lice, Pediculosis hominis var. corporis causes body lice, and Pthirus pubis causes pubic lice, also known as "crabs." These small insects are just a few millimeters in size, but can be seen with the naked eye if you look closely for them. The lice lay eggs, which are called nits, and are also visible with the naked eye.

Head lice are commonly seen in children, and outbreaks frequently occur in schools and day care centers. Interestingly, children of African descent are less likely to get head lice, perhaps because of the shape of the tightly curled hair shaft. These infestations are sometimes, but not always, itchy. The nits that adhere to the hair can look like dandruff at first glance but are not removed as easily as dandruff would be. To see if you or your child has head lice, you can run a fine-toothed comb through the hair, starting at the root. If present, lice and nits are visible in the comb.

Body lice do not actually live on the body, instead they live on clothing. They can survive for up to a month before taking their next feeding on a human host. Itching is the main symptom that you will experience if you have body lice. Check the seams of your clothes and bed linens to identify the insects and their nits.

Pubic lice live within the pubic hairs on their human host. Like body lice, crabs are very itchy. They are usually sexually transmitted and are not prevented by use of a condom. Occasionally

Examine the scalp and hair closely to check for head lice and their nits.

pubic lice can also be found in the underarms or in the eyelashes. Over-the-counter and prescription medications containing the active ingredients permethrin, pyrethrin, and malathion are available to treat lice. Lindane is considered a second-line treatment.

Lichen planus

Lichen planus is a common rash that can affect the skin, mouth, genitals, nails, or the scalp. It is often described by the six p's: pruritic (itchy), polygonal, planar (flat-topped), purple papules (small raised bumps) and plaques (large raised bumps). This condition routinely lasts for several months, and may wax and wane during that time. It usually burns out within 18 months, but some people find that it flares even years after the initial eruption. While the cause of this condition is not known, it is sometimes seen as a reaction to medication, or in association with a hepatitis C infection.

Usually lichen planus is a harmless eruption that is a nuisance. However, erosive forms that leave the skin with open wounds can be quite painful. This form occurs most commonly in the mouth. Lichen planus may be treated with topical steroids, tacrolimus, light treatments, oral steroids, oral retinoids, immune suppressants, hydroxychloroquine, or dapsone.

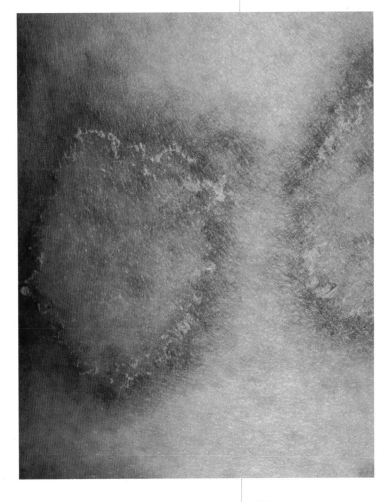

Lupus has different rashes associated with the acute, subacute cutaneous, and chronic forms of the disease.

Lupus

Lupus is an autoimmune disease where the body acts against itself to cause swelling, inflammation, and tissue destruction. Lupus of the skin is divided into three categories. Acute cutaneous lupus (ACL) is characterized by a "butterfly rash" over the cheeks along with photosensitivity. ACL is closely associated with systemic lupus, which commonly involves the lungs, joints, heart, kidney, liver, and brain, among other organs. Subacute cutaneous lupus (SCLE) is characterized by a pink or red, slightly scaly eruption that comes and goes. This condition is sensitive to the sun and may also be exacerbated by some medications. It does not leave scars when it goes away.

Some patients with SCLE also have systemic lupus. Chronic cutaneous lupus, or discoid lupus, may be seen in patients with systemic lupus, but most often it is seen in patients without other forms of lupus. These spots may be pink, red, or purple scaly lesions on the face or scalp. These spots heal with scarring. If you suspect that you have lupus, you should see your doctor. Go to your visit prepared with a complete list of your medications, because there are several that can cause lupus. Your doctor might check some blood work and might perform a biopsy in order to help make a diagnosis. While lupus is a chronic condition, treatments are available both for skin involvement and for systemic involvement to try to keep this condition under control.

> Hair loss occurs in almost half of lupus patients at some point during their disease.

Melanocytic nevi

Commonly referred to as moles, melanocytic nevi may be present from birth or develop any time during the course of one's lifetime. Congenital nevi are categorized as small, medium, or large. These moles may have hair growing from them. They grow as you grow, and they might become more raised off the skin surface over time. It is important to know that congenital nevi do have the risk of developing into melanoma skin cancer. The risk is greatest with the large congenital nevi and smallest with the small congenital nevi. You should discuss the risks, benefits, and timing of excision of these moles with your dermatologist.

> Examine your moles regularly to monitor for changes in size, shape, and color.

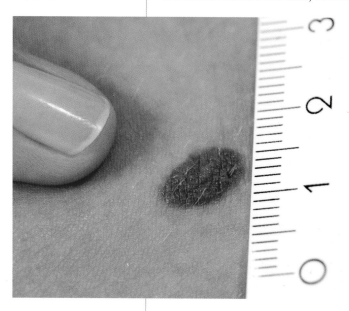

Acquired nevi can develop any time after birth. Moles may be flesh colored, tan, or brown. They sometimes start out flat and become more raised as we get older. They also sometimes lose their color, starting out tan or brown, but becoming more flesh colored over time. It is important that you let a professional evaluate any moles you have that are changing, even though not all changes are bad.

Some moles just don't look quite right. They are funny looking. Your doctor might call them atypical or dysplastic. She will likely want to perform a biopsy in order to evaluate them under the microscope. Information obtained from the microscopic examination that your doctor will evaluate can be quite complex. What is important for you to know is that your doctor will make a recommendation about whether the biopsy was sufficient or whether the mole needs to be re-excised after the initial interpretation of the biopsy. While atypical nevi are still benign, they do pose an increased risk of developing into melanoma in the future. Also people who have multiple atypical nevi are at increased risk for developing melanoma. Everyone should have a full-body skin exam by a medical professional each year to minimize the risk of developing skin cancer and to identify and treat skin cancers as early as possible.

CONGENITAL NEVI	
Type	Size
Small	Less than 2 cm
Medium	2–20 cm
Large	Greater than 20 cm

Melasma

Have you ever heard of the "mask of pregnancy"? That is a common name for the condition whose proper name is melasma. This disease is frequently seen in women who have extra estrogen in their systems, mainly from being pregnant or from taking birth control pills.

However, just because you have melasma does not mean that you have high estrogen levels, and many women who get melasma are not pregnant and do not take oral contraceptives. Melasma is particularly common in women of African, Asian and Middle Eastern descent, and Latinas, but people of any ethnic background may suffer from it. Men get melasma less frequently than women do.

How do you know if you have melasma? It is characterized by a tan, brown, or grayish-brown discoloration of the skin. It usually occurs on the face but may also appear on the chest or arms. The forehead, cheeks, upper lip and chin are the most common areas involved. The borders of the discoloration are usually irregular rather than being smooth. Many people notice that their melasma is worse in the summer; that is because sunlight makes it darker and more noticeable.

Melasma can occur in anyone, but it is most common in women who are pregnant, on birth control pills, or hormone replacement therapy, and women with richly pigmented skin.

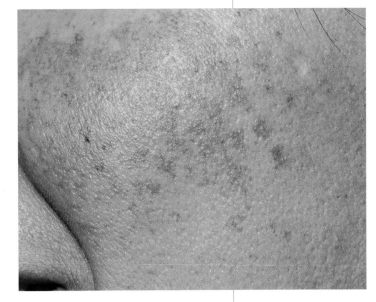

There are several different ways to treat melasma. Everyone with this condition needs to wear sunscreen faithfully. You should look for products containing an SPF of 30 or higher with broad spectrum UVA and UVB protection.

Over-the-counter fade creams containing hydroquinone are often not strong enough to manage this condition, but may be tried before seeking the help of a dermatologist. A doctor will probably offer a prescription of a higher concentration hydroquinone cream and may add a second medication, such as a topical retinoid. Chemical peels are usually very effective in speeding up the fading of the discoloration. Lasers are also helpful in treating this pigmentation, but because they are more expensive than topical medications and chemical peels, they are usually reserved for more severe or resistant cases.

If you are taking birth control pills, you may need to have a conversation with your doctor about alternative forms of contraception because it can be difficult to clear melasma if you remain on the pill. If you are pregnant, you should wait until after delivery and breast-feeding before beginning treatment for this condition.

Milia

Milia are tiny cysts that appear on the face. They are usually just one or two millimeters in size. They may look like a closed comedone, also called a whitehead, or even like a pustule. No matter how hard you try, these lesions cannot be removed by just squeezing them out. Of course, you should not try to squeeze any spots on your face! When they occur in children, milia usually resolve on their own. In adults they do not just go away, but they are easily extracted by a dermatologist. The surface of the skin is nicked with a scalpel. Then a comedone extractor is used to remove the contents.

Molluscum contagiosum

If you have children, then you may have heard of molluscum contagiousum, often just called molluscum. Molluscum is a common condition and is caused by a poxvirus. Each molluscum lesion is a

SKIN SOLUTION

To prevent melasma from worsening or recurring, it is important to wear sunscreen every day, all year long. Look for products with broad spectrum coverage, including **UVA** and **UVB** protection, and an **SPF** of at least 30. Corrective cosmetics can be used to conceal the dark areas and often contain sunscreens that will also help protect the skin.

Milia commonly occurs on the face but can also appear on the groin.

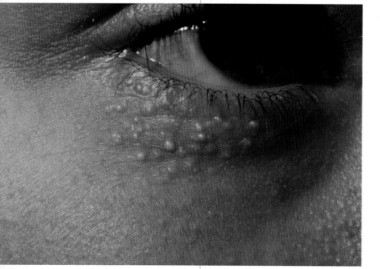

small, flesh-colored papule with a central indentation. This is called an umbilication because it dents in like an umbilicus (belly button). Lesions vary in size but usually range from 1 to 5 millimeters. You may have just one, but more often there are several lesions, sometimes dozens, at a time. Molluscum is usually found in children and sometimes in child-care providers. The lesions can occur anywhere on the body, including the chest, arms, legs, or face. This disease can also occur in young adults; it is often sexually transmitted and can occur in the groin. Molluscum contagiosum is also seen in people whose immune systems are compromised by medication or by diseases such as HIV. Left untreated, molluscum usually resolves on its own.

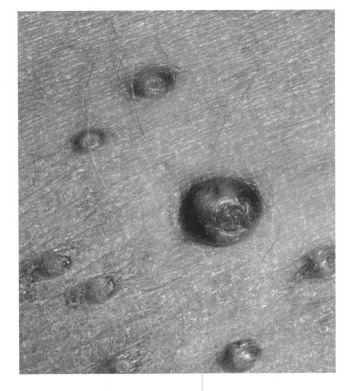

These dimpled lesions, seen here on the skin of a 12-year-old girl, are caused by a molluscum contagiosum virus infection.

However, this resolution usually takes several months, even up to a year. Because the condition is contagious, it is often advisable to treat the spots to prevent them from spreading elsewhere on the body or from getting passed on to someone else. A doctor can often diagnose molluscum just by looking at the skin. Occasionally a biopsy is needed to confirm the diagnosis because there are less common conditions that can sometimes look similar to molluscum, particularly in immuno-compromised patients. Several treatment options are available. Cantharadin is a common medication that a physician applies to the spots. It is derived from the blister beetle and may cause irritation or even a blister at the site of application. Sometimes the lesions are scraped off with an instrument called a curette. And sometimes a medication intended for other purposes, such as tretinoin, may cause mild to severe irritation of the skin. Molluscum lesions may take several treatments before complete resolution is achieved.

The molluscum lesions will resolve on their own over a period of several months or more, but it is possible to spread the infection.

Pityriasis rosea

This harmless rash usually occurs in people between the ages of 10 and 35. You might first notice the "herald patch," a single, pink or salmon-colored spot that is several centimeters in diameter. Shortly thereafter, several similar smaller lesions erupt on the back, chest, abdomen, groin, arms, or legs. The spots tend to have a slightly raised edge and are a

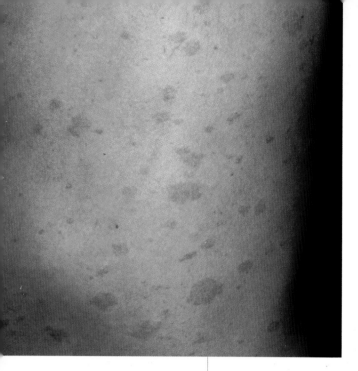

lighter pink in the center where there is usually a fine white scale. In people with brown skin, the individual spots may be tan or brown rather than pink. Doctors don't know what causes this condition, but we think it may be caused by a virus. This condition usually clears on its own after approximately two months, although occasionally it can last longer.

Pityriasis rosea is usually asymptomatic, but a physician may prescribe topical steroids, ultraviolet light, or antihistamines if the skin itches.

Poison ivy

Would you recognize the poison ivy plant if you saw it? Its three-pointed leaf is easily recognizable to many of those who garden or hike. The problem is that the telltale leaf is often not noticed until it has come into contact with the skin. The plant produces a substance called urushiol, which is a skin irritant. This toxic substance causes redness, swelling, and even blistering in the areas it touches. And, as anyone who has suffered from poison ivy knows, it is very, very itchy. Poison ivy is, in fact, a form of irritant contact dermatitis.

Prevention is best when it comes to poison ivy. If you plan to be outside in

Pityriasis rosea starts with one large pink spot, the "herald patch," which is followed by the characteristic rash of smaller spots, usually on the chest and back.

LEFT: The characteristic leaflets of poison ivy are the cause of the common warning, "Leaves of three, let them be!"

RIGHT: Poison ivy exposure is characterized by an intensely itchy red rash with blisters. Antihistamines and topical, or oral corticosteroids help to relieve the symptoms.

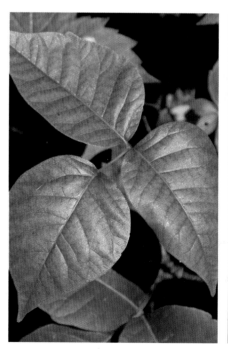

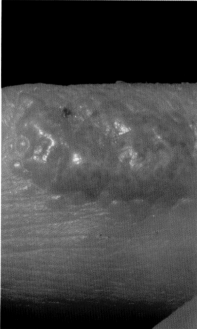

an area where the plant may be present, protective clothing is very helpful. Long trousers and socks are useful while hiking, and gloves are important for gardeners. If you believe that you have come into contact with poison ivy, you should wash the area of contact immediately with hot or cold water. Mild eruptions can be treated with over-the-counter hydrocortisone cream. If the rash is extensive, then prescription-strength topical steroids may be needed to help clear the rash and keep you comfortable.

A doctor may prescribe oral steroids for very severe cases of poison ivy.

Psoriasis

Have you ever heard of the "heartbreak of psoriasis"? Most people with psoriasis are otherwise healthy, but this condition can affect your quality of life. Psoriasis patients are often very self-conscious, and some people alter their lives to accommodate their disease.

The cause of psoriasis is not well understood. Many patients have a genetic predisposition, and the condition seems to be a malfunctioning of the immune system. It is characterized by a raised pink rash with a silvery scale. The scale is said to resemble mica, which also has a silvery quality. It is commonly found on the scalp, elbows, knees, and buttocks, but it can occur anywhere on the body. A person often has several areas of rash at a time, and each spot may range in size from a centimeter to entire areas of the body.

Psoriasis can occur anywhere on the body and most commonly involves the skin of the elbows, knees, scalp, and buttocks.

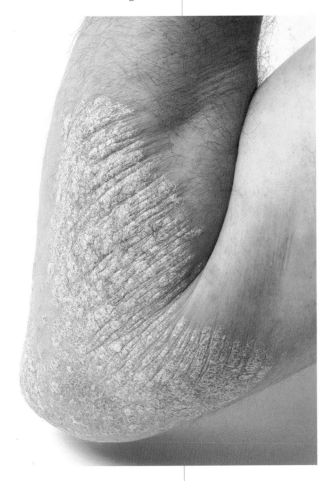

There are different types of psoriasis. In guttate psoriasis, the individual spots are all small, just a few centimeters. This condition is often preceded by an infection. Patients with pustular psoriasis are covered in pustules and are often quite ill.

Unfortunately, there is no cure for psoriasis, but it can be managed. If you suspect that you have psoriasis, you should see a dermatologist. You may be given topical steroids or vitamin D medication such as calcipotriene or you may be treated with light therapy. People with severe psoriasis may be treated with oral medications that suppress the immune system. Recently there has emerged a new class of medication called the biologics. These include etanercept (Enbrel), alefacept (Amevive), adalimumab (Humira), infliximab (Remicade), and ustekinumab (Stelara).

PUPPP

Pruritic urticarial papules and plaques of pregnancy (PUPPP) is one of the most common skin rashes seen in pregnant women. This eruption usually occurs in the third trimester of a woman's first pregnancy and is extremely itchy. The rash usually begins on the abdomen and extends to the arms, legs, and back but does not generally involve the face, palms, or soles. On the abdomen, it tends to be found within the stretch marks, but it spares the belly button area. This umbilical sparing is a key feature that helps to distinguish PUPPP from a much less common disease of pregnancy called pemphigoid gestationis (formerly called herpes gestationis). Your obstetrician may send you to a dermatologist to help make this distinction.

The PUPPP rash is made of small or large pink bumps, or hivelike spots, or even small water blisters, called vesicles. The cause of this condition is not known, but it is interesting that the majority of women who develop PUPPP give birth to boys and many of the affected women are carrying multiples. The "cure" for this rash is delivery, after which it usually resolves within a week or so. Other than that, very itchy cases may be treated with topical steroid medicines prescribed by your doctor. Very severe cases might be treated with oral antihistamines to help control the itch as well as steroids by mouth to control the rash. Women who develop PUPPP during one pregnancy do not usually develop the condition during subsequent pregnancies.

SKIN SOLUTION

Giving birth is the best treatment for **PUPPP**, which usually resolves shortly after delivery. In the meantime, stay comfortable with cool baths and anti-itch lotions.

The rash of PUPPP frequently begins in the stretch marks of the abdomen and can also spread to the thighs, breasts, and arms.

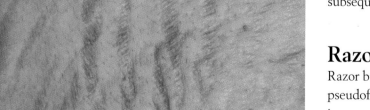

Razor bumps

Razor bumps are also called pseudofolliculitis barbae. This condition is commonly seen in the beard area in men. It also occurs in women who grow hairs on the chin, jaw, or neck, and in women who shave the bikini area. It is most common in people with curly, coarse hair. So, it is seen disproportionately in people of African descent, but it can occur in all ethnicities. The curled hair may pierce the hair follicle wall while it is growing inside the follicle, before it ever reaches the surface of the skin. Or the hair may grow beyond the skin's surface, curl around and pierce the skin's surface from the outside. Either way, the hair then causes an inflammation of the follicle and bumps result.

The best way to manage razor bumps is to avoid growing hair. This can be achieved with laser hair removal, electrolysis, or with the prescription cream eflornithine. Razor bumps may also be treated with acne treatments medications, such as benzoyl peroxide, retinoids, or topical antibiotics. Some people find that changing their method of hair removal can decrease the incidence of razor bumps. Depilatories soften the hair and decrease their ability to pierce the skin.

Some men find that using an electric clipper or a foil guard razor is a good option to avoid a shave that is too close. Others prefer triple or quadruple blade manual razors. Ultimately some men must simply grow a beard to avoid developing these lesions.

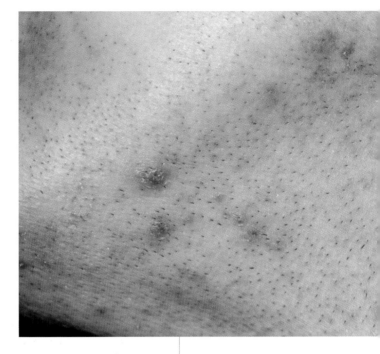

Pseudofolliculitis barbae is most commonly seen on the male face, but it can also occur on other parts of the body where hair is shaved or plucked.

Rosacea

Have you ever been told that you have a rosy glow? If redness on the apples of your cheeks waxes and wanes or persists, you may have rosacea. Formerly known as acne rosacea, this condition is very common. It is seen more often in women than in men. There are four main variants. Early on, you may experience the first symptom of flushing and blushing. This gives the cheeks or whole face a rosy appearance. Each person has her own triggers, but the usual ones are caffeine, alcohol, spicy food, and exercise. The redness may be transient or persistent.

A second form of rosacea is the "papulopustular" form. With this you might have pink pimples or pus-filled bumps on the face. This eruption is sometimes confused with acne. Rhynophyma, the third form, is seen particularly in men. The sebaceous glands of the nose enlarge, causing the nose itself to enlarge and sometimes change its shape. Finally, rosacea can involve the eyes. If you have rosacea and experience a sensation of dry eyes, you should see an ophthalmologist to determine if your eyes are affected. The treatment for rosacea depends on which form you have. For the redness

Skin Myth

True or False?
Rosacea is caused by drinking too much alcohol.

False

In fact the exact cause of rosacea is unknown. There are many things that can make it flare up, including spicy foods, caffeine, exercise, hot beverages and alcohol, but these are not the cause of the disease.

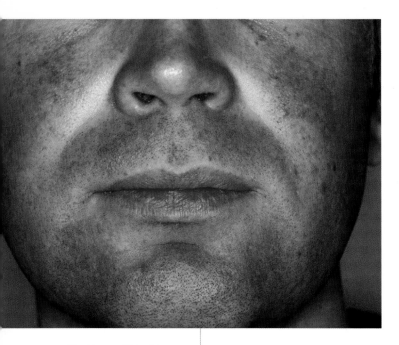

of flushing, there are several over-the-counter preparations (see Redness section, page 51). A physician may prescribe a sulfur-containing wash, topical metronidazole, topical azeleic acid, oral antibiotics, or a combination of these medications for the papules and pustules. In addition to these prescription medications, chemical peels may be useful in controlling the symptoms. Rhynophyma can be improved by reshaping the nose using an ablative laser or by electrocautery. This procedure should be performed only by a skin, plastic, or ENT surgeon experienced in the procedure.

Flushing and blushing are often the first signs of rosacea. Other signs are papules, pustules, nose enlargement called rhynophyma, and eye involvement.

BELOW: Scabies mites burrow in the stratum corneum, the uppermost layer of the epidermis, where they lay their eggs.

Scabies

Scabies infection is caused by the sarcoptes scabiei mite. It is also known as mange and the seven-year itch. The mite is so small that it is not visible to the naked eye. However, the mite tunnels beneath the uppermost layer of the skin, and those burrows are easily seen. You will see white straight or curvy lines a few millimeters long. In addition, red bumps or even small blisters may be seen. The rash occurs usually in the finger and toe-web spaces, belly button, waist, and groin, but it may occur anywhere on the body. Scabies causes people to be very, very itchy.

It is highly contagious and is passed easily from person to person by skin contact. For this reason it frequently affects children and people living in close quarters, such as nursing homes. The condition may be particularly severe in the elderly and in people who are immuno-compromised.

Permethrin is the treatment of choice for treating scabies. Lindane or malathion can also be used. These preparations are applied from the neck down and left in place overnight before being washed off. This treatment is usually repeated in a week. For severe cases, ivermectin may be given orally.

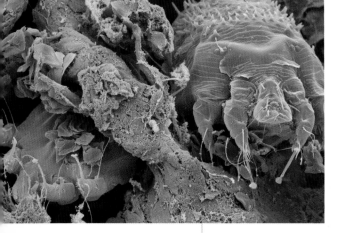

Sebaceous hyperplasia

You may not have realized that you can actually see enlarged oil glands (sebaceous hyperplasia) on the surface of your skin. These glands appear on the forehead, nose, or cheeks of individuals with particularly oily skin. The enlarged glands have a characteristic yellow-pink color and a depressed or umbilicated center; they are soft to the touch and are a few millimeters in size. There may be one or multiple lesions.

Removal is unnecessary, as there is no cancerous potential, but it can be easily done for cosmetic reasons. The methods of removal can include "burning" with an electric needle (electro-cautery), freezing with liquid nitrogen, treating with chemicals such as trichloracetic acid, or cutting with a surgical blade, scissor, or laser. Complications could include scarring or, for individuals with darker skin tones, long-lasting light or dark discoloration.

Sebaceous hyperplasia occurs more often in middle age, and more men have sebaceous hyperplasia than women.

Skin cancer

Because of the importance of skin cancer and its treatment on your overall well-being, skin cancers are discussed in detail in chapter 5.

Skin tags

Skin tags are extra pieces of skin that occur on the neck and under the arms and breasts. They often protrude from the surface of the skin and appear attached to the skin by a thin stalk. Skin tags are harmless. They do not become cancerous but can easily become irritated when rubbed by jewelry, clothing, or seatbelts. Skin tags develop more readily during pregnancy, if you are overweight, and as you mature. Skin tags may bleed if traumatized, turn black if twisted, or fall off if irritated. Since they are benign, treatment is not required. But if they bother you, they can easily be removed.

An old-fashioned home remedy is to tie a string around the skin tag. This cuts off the blood supply of the tag, and it will fall off after several days. Since the area may become red and tender during the process, it is best to see a physician for removal. Your doctor may remove the tag using a surgical scissor to snip

Skin tags should not be confused with moles because they are made of completely different cells.

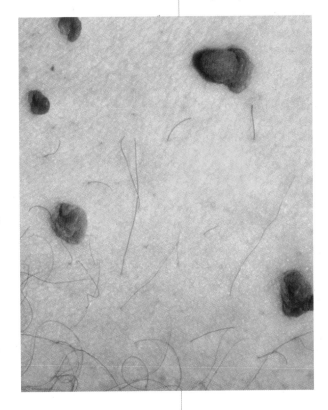

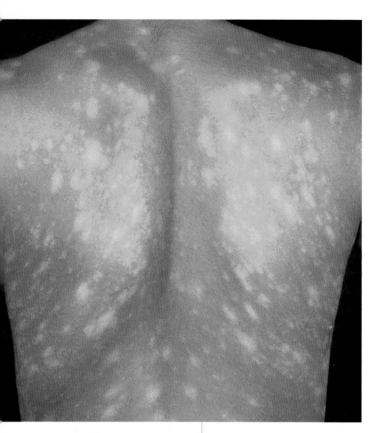

The discoloration caused by tinea versicolor is more apparent if the skin becomes tanned.

it off, an electric needle (electrocautery) to "burn" the tag off, or liquid nitrogen to freeze it. Although freezing skin tags with liquid nitrogen is an acceptable treatment for lighter skin types, it is riskier for darker skin types because it can lead to light or dark marks.

Tinea versicolor

Tinea versicolor, also known as pityriasis versicolor, is a rash caused by a superficial infection of the skin with a fungus called Malassezia furfur. While words like "pityriasis" and "Malassezia" may sound scary, this is actually a very common and totally harmless rash seen most commonly in teens and young adults. It usually occurs on the chest, back, and arms, and sometimes on the face. It is seen in the spring and summer months, or year-round in warmer climates. It may appear tan, pink, or brown and usually has a fine white scale that is particularly noticeable if you scratch it. The condition is sometimes itchy. Tinea versicolor is usually flat or slightly raised, and individual circular spots may be seen or large areas of skin may be covered. Sometimes as the condition resolves, there are light spots that are left behind on the skin that can take several weeks or months to fade. Tinea versicolor is usually easily diagnosed by its appearance, and your physician may take a skin scraping to confirm the diagnosis. It is effectively treated by prescription topical antifungal medications, but oral antifungal pills are sometimes needed for a more extensive disease.

SKIN SOLUTION

Some people suffer from tinea versicolor every spring. Talk to your doctor about using prescription-strength selenium-sulfide shampoo weekly as a preventive measure.

Varicella

Varicella (chicken pox) is a common disease of childhood. Its symptoms are fever, muscle aches, and malaise followed by a rash. The rash consists of small water blisters surrounded by red skin. These spots usually start on the head and neck, then spread down to the trunk. The lower body may be affected but is often spared. This uncomfortable, itchy rash usually persists for 7 to 10 days.

Varicella is contagious and is spread through respiratory droplets and direct contact with the rash. A person is contagious for 5 to 7 days before the rash appears and then until all of the little blisters have crusted over. This disease can be quite serious in adults, pregnant women, and those who are immuno-compromised.

Mild cases of varicella can be managed with acetaminophen to reduce fever and antihistamines to reduce itch. However, it is advisable to see a physician early in the course of the disease. If the rash is treated within the first 3 days, antiviral medications can shorten its course. The most common complication of varicella is bacterial infection of the skin, but more serious side effects can occur. The varicella vaccine is a live attenuated virus. It is available in several counties throughout the world, though guidelines for administration vary from country to country. Mobidity and mortality from varicella have decreased in countries where the vaccine is routinely used.

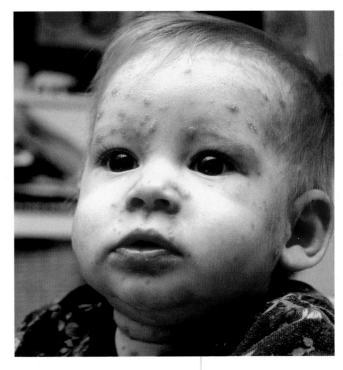

Chicken pox is a highly contagious disease that is common in children. It is more severe in adults.

Vitiligo

Vitiligo is a condition in which the skin loses its pigmentation, causing white spots in small or large areas. These white spots are more evident in people with richly pigmented skin or in the spring and summer months, when light skin acquires a suntan. It is impossible to predict the course of the disease: for some it spreads very slowly, but for others it moves very quickly and affects large areas of the body.

Complicated genetic factors appear to play a role in the transmission of vitilgo, but its cause is still not clear. Skin affected by vitiligo loses functional melanocytes, which normally produce the skin's pigment. Among treatments for vitiligo are topical medicines, light treatment, lasers, and occasionally surgical procedures. Camouflage cosmetics can be used to conceal areas of depigmentation caused by vitiligo. Appropriate medicines include topical steroids and topical immuno-supressants. Repigmentation may also be achieved by using light treatment. Narrow-band UVB is most commonly used, but PUVA (Psoralen and UVA treatment) is also used. This treatment should be performed under a physician's

SKIN SOLUTION

Camouflage cosmetics can be used to conceal areas of depigmentation caused by vitiligo. These products offer better coverage, are longer lasting than regular makeup products, and are formulated for use anywhere on the body.

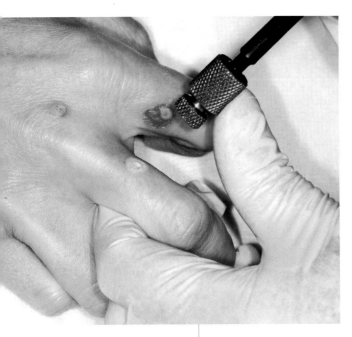

Liquid nitrogen cryotherapy is often used to treat warts.

supervision. You should not go to a tanning center in an attempt to treat vitiligo yourself. Some doctors treat vitiligo with the excimer laser with good success. Others will graft pigmented skin in to areas with vitiligo.

In rare instances, a person may have lost so much pigment that it is better to eliminate the remaining pigment than to attempt to bring back what has been lost. In this case, a medication called monobenzyl ether of hydroquinone may be prescribed to achieve this goal.

Warts

Warts are found in both children and adults. They are caused by a group of viruses called the human papillomaviruses (HPV) and are easily spread from person to person by casual contact. There are many types of warts because there are hundreds of HPVs. Some viruses prefer the surface of the skin, others prefer the palms of the hands and soles of the feet, while still others prefer mucosal surfaces such as the mouth or the genitals.

Common warts are dome-shaped papules with an uneven surface that often appears dry or crusty. They usually occur on the hands or at sites of trauma, such as the knee. Flat warts look very different and are sometimes hard to see. They are very thin growths that sometimes have a pink appearance. They are usually found on the face and the back of the hands. Palmar and plantar warts occur on the palms of the hands and the soles of the feet. Rather than protruding from the surface of the skin like common warts, they often exist below the surface. Condyloma acuminata occur in the genital or anal area and can be sexually transmitted.

If left untreated, warts sometimes resolve by themselves. However, this usually takes a year or more; and in that time, warts can spread to other parts of your body or to other people.

There are many over-the-counter wart medications. Salicylic acid preparations and freezing methods are readily available. Many people have also had success with covering the wart with duct tape and filing it with an emery board or pumice stone every few days.

Warts that do not respond to over-the-counter treatments can be treated by a physician. There are treatment options: freezing with liquid nitrogen; cutting the wart off; application of an acid preparation; electrosurgery; or laser surgery. Condyloma acuminate may be treated in the doctor's office with a topical medication called podophyllin or at home with a topical-prescription medication called imiquimod. Your doctor should discuss the

Skin Myth

True or False?
Warts have roots.

False

In fact warts are a viral infection of the epidermis, the uppermost layer of the skin. Even large warts do not have roots that extend deep into lower layers of the skin. They can be difficult to treat and sometimes recur because the wart virus is resilient, not because warts have roots.

best option for you. This depends on your skin type and the location and size of the wart.

Zoster

Zoster is known by several names. It is also called herpes zoster and shingles. This condition is caused by the varicella zoster virus. Most people are infected with this virus in childhood and develop the skin condition varicella, or chicken pox (see page 105). Once you are infected, the virus never leaves your body. It lives in the nerves for several decades without causing any trouble. Later in life, usually in the 50s or later, the virus can become active again and cause a new rash.

Unlike varicella, which can affect the whole body, zoster usually affects one area of the body, and follows skin lines called dermatomes. The rash consists of tiny water blisters, called vesicles, similar to those of varicella. The skin surrounding these water blisters is usually red and the eruption is characterized by significant pain. The rash usually clears up within one to two weeks, but the pain may persist for several weeks.

Zoster will cause you the least discomfort if you begin medical treatment as soon as possible, ideally within the first 72 hours. This can shorten the duration of both the eruption and the pain. The effective medications are acyclovir, valacyclovir, and famcyclovir. There are also several options for managing the associated pain, and these should be discussed with your doctor.

In order to reduce the likelihood of developing shingles, people aged 60 and over should be immunized with the zoster vaccine. The vaccine works best in people aged 60–69, where it reduces the rate of shingles by 50 percent. Older patients also have a decreased risk of developing shingles after being vaccinated, but the effectiveness decreases with age. People who have weakened immune systems, people with tuberculosis that have not been treated, pregnant women, and people who are allergic to neomycin or gelatin should not receive the vaccine.

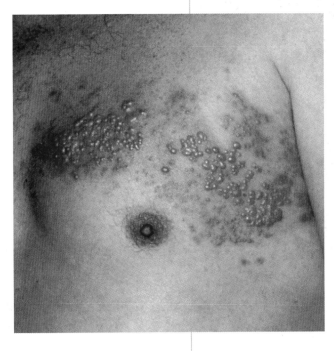

The unilateral, linear, painful rash is characteristic of zoster.

4

Cosmetic and Surgical Procedures

In today's society images of models who are the perfect height, weight, proportion, and size surround us in magazines, newspapers, TV programs, and the Internet. The perceived "perfect face" is smooth and soft with luscious lips, a straight nose, and without a hint of any discolorations, wrinkles, or breakouts. Alas, these people do not represent the real world, and we would be wise to remember that.

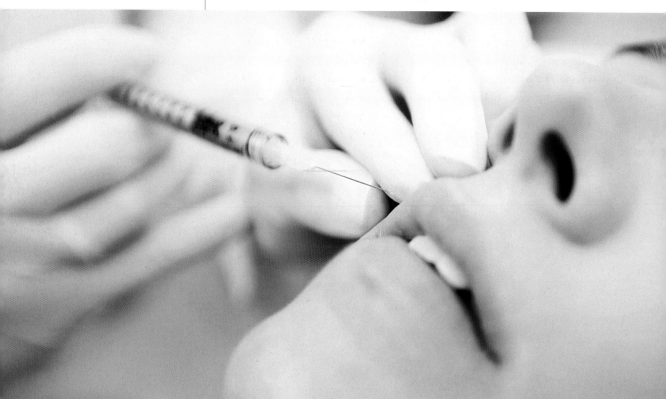

The good, the bad, and the ugly

In reality, no one's appearance is perfect. And it is our individual variation that makes each of us beautiful and special. While we may not have the same team of professionals available to movie stars, a lot about our appearance actually is under our control. Taking care of yourself is reflected in a better appearance, and you don't need a personal trainer and chef to eat well and exercise.

The last two decades have seen tremendous advancements in the technology available to improve the appearance of your skin. The number of procedures, products, and devices that are available to enhance appearance without invasive surgery has actually outpaced traditional cosmetic surgery. Even the surgeries have improved, and many have become less invasive. The cost for many of these procedures has decreased, making them accessible to more and more people.

Self-esteem

Before starting down the path of cosmetic enhancement, it is very important that you assess your motivations honestly. Cosmetic procedures and surgeries can improve your appearance. They will not change your life or who you are as a person. It is important to have a positive, healthy sense of who you are before you seek cosmetic treatment. Most people would agree that the best cosmetic treatments do not significantly change your looks. They may make you look fresher, less tired, or a few years younger.

Cosmetic procedures that dramatically alter your features are usually considered extreme, and look odd. Because well-performed procedures are not going to transform you into a new person, it is very important to be happy with who you are before you start down this path. For some people this may even require therapy. Seeking help for any issues you have about your identity, appearance, or self-esteem is a very positive step.

Skin Myth

True or False?
Body dysmorphic disorder is an illness that causes people to become preoccupied with minor or non-existent flaws.

True

SYMPTOMS OF BDD

Seek professional advice if you suspect that someone you know is showing signs of the following symptoms:

- Being preoccupied with minor or imaginary physical flaws
- Having a lot of anxiety about the perceived flaw and spending a lot of time focusing on it
- Repeatedly checking appearance in a mirror
- Hiding minor imperfections
- Comparing appearance with others
- Excessively grooming
- Seeking reassurance from others about how they look

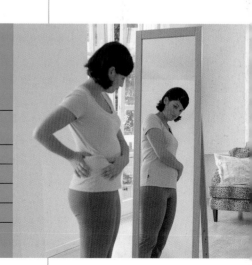

Body dysmorphic disorder (BDD) is an illness. It causes people to be preoccupied with minor or non-existent "flaws" in their appearance. This preoccupation can take up several hours a day and can make it hard to focus on the normal activities of everyday life or have normal social interactions.

There are several characteristic behaviors that people with BDD may exhibit. These may include a lot of time spent in front of the mirror, use of heavy makeup, or obsessive-compulsive habits such as skin picking or hair pulling. Some people with BDD avoid social situations, avoid taking pictures, or even avoid looking in mirrors because they are so disturbed by their appearance.

While BDD affects approximately 1 percent of the population, approximately 10 percent of people seeking cosmetic surgery are affected. A good doctor will screen for this disorder before agreeing to perform an elective procedure or surgery. These patients often undergo multiple procedures but are never satisfied. If this condition reminds you of someone you know, or if you think you may have BDD, it is important to recognize that this condition is treatable. Many people have been helped with psychotherapy, medication, or a combination of the two. Treatment should be sought from a board-certified psychiatrist.

> BDD is not an incurable condition. In fact, therapy by a trained psychiatrist or psychologist, as well as prescribed medications, will likely result in long-lasting improvement.

Choosing wisely

While most cosmetic procedures and surgeries are performed safely and with good results, it is important to know that every treatment has risks and potential side effects. It is important for you to try to minimize those risks and side effects. How can you do this? There are several steps that you can take.

It is important to select a good doctor. A recommendation from another doctor you trust or from a friend who had a good experience is the best way to find a doctor. You may want to have consultations with more than one doctor before you make a selection. Ask to see before and after photos of other patients they have treated, and ask about their experience in performing the procedure that you are interested in. You should ask if the doctor is board-certified, and if so, in what field. You would not go to an orthopedic surgeon for your annual Pap smear. Likewise, your cosmetic procedures and surgeries should be entrusted to specialists like dermatologists, plastic surgeons, otorhinolaringologists (ear, nose, and throat doctors) and ophthalmologists.

QUESTIONS TO ASK YOUR SURGEON

- Can I see before and after photos of other patients?

- How much experience have you had in this particular procedure?

- What are your success rates for this operation?

- What is the rate of complications that you experience with this kind of operation?

Cosmetic procedures

You do not have to undergo surgery to achieve younger looking skin. There are plenty of non-surgical treatments available.

Chemical peels

A chemical peel involves the application of an acid to the surface of the skin. The purpose of this application is to create a controlled destruction of the uppermost layers of the skin in order to speed up the generation of new, healthier skin. As such, chemical peels offer superficial skin resurfacing that improves the texture and appearance of the skin.

Chemical peels are effective in the management of several different skin conditions. They are commonly used to treat photodamaged skin. The fine lines, sunspots (solar lentigos), and even the actinic keratoses that result from chronic sun exposure can all be improved with chemical peels.

Acne patients also do very well with chemical peels for several reasons. Peels can help unclog the pores. Because they are drying to the skin, the peels also create an environment that is less hospitable for the bacteria that cause the acne. Peels can also hasten the fading of the dark spots that are left after a pimple resolves; this is called post-inflammatory hyperpigmentation, or PIH.

In addition to treating PIH from acne, chemical peels can be used to treat other forms of pigmentation. For instance, people with melasma or PIH from other conditions can be treated effectively. Peels can also improve rosacea, help to manage oily skin, and improve the appearance of small scars.

Chemical peels are classified by how deep into the skin they work. Superficial peels work in the epidermis only. Medium-depth chemical peels treat the epidermis and the papillary dermis. Deep peels extend well into the dermis. There are two factors that dictate whether a peel is superficial, medium, or deep. The first is which acid is used, and the second is the strength, or concentration, of that acid.

The decisions of which peel to use and at what strength depend on your skin type, the condition being treated, and how sensitive your skin is.

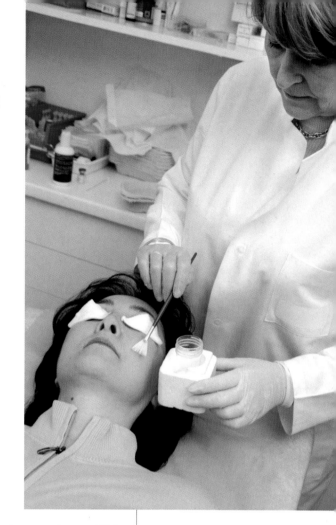

When a chemical peel is applied to the skin, it removes the upper most layers revealing new, radiant skin beneath.

When carried out by a professional who is well trained in performing the procedure, chemical peels can lead to smooth, soft, and even-toned skin.

A superficial chemical peel will remove the stratum corneum (top pink layer) and a portion of the epidermis (darker pink layer underneath).

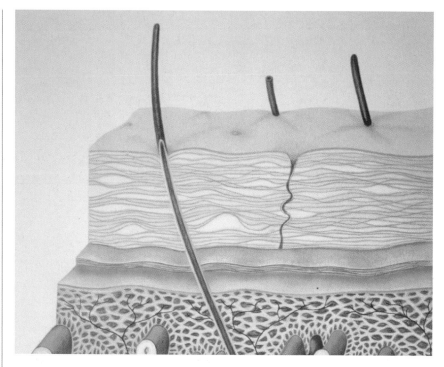

Many doctors will pre-treat the skin for several days or weeks before a chemical peel. Agents like sunscreens, retinoids, or bleaching agents may be prescribed alone or in combination. All three help to reduce the risk of post-inflammatory hyperpigmentation after the peel. This is of particular concern for people with olive or brown skin tones. In addition, if a medium or deep peel is performed and you are prone to developing cold sores from herpes simplex virus, you may be put on antiviral pills, such as acyclovir, valacyclovir, or famcyclovir.

SKIN SOLUTION

There are several different agents that may be selected for your chemical peel, including glycolic acid, salicylic acid, trichloroacetic acid, or lactic acid.

What can you expect when you go for a chemical peel? First the skin will be cleansed. You can make this step easier and more effective by not wearing makeup to your appointment. A primer may then be applied to the skin. This primer may be alcohol or acetone, and it may also contain a lower level of the acid that will be applied during the peel. The peeling agent is applied to the skin, often with a cotton swab, gauze, or on a pre-soaked pad. Depending on the acid and strength used, you may experience anything from light tingling to a burning sensation. This should be discussed with your doctor in advance.

Some peels require the step of neutralizing the acid to get it to stop working. Other acids do not require neutralization because they stop working on their own. Most peels are left on between three and five minutes before they self-neutralize or are neutralized by the doctor.

After a superficial chemical peel, the skin is often blotchy and red. The skin may also feel dry and be flaky for a few days. Usually the skin returns to normal between one and three days. Medium-depth peels often leave the skin feeling raw. Redness may persist for several days, and there is usually more significant desquamation (peeling). After a medium-depth peel, the skin usually returns to normal after five to seven days. Deep chemical peels are seldom used now. Laser treatments are usually preferable to deep chemical peels, especially for the treatment of problems involving the texture of the skin. Recent advances have made the effects of the laser more consistent and controllable, particularly when disruption of the dermal layer of the skin is required to bring about the desired improvement in the skin.

CHEMICAL PEELS	
Type of peel	**Use**
Superficial	Requires minimal recovery time as the most superficial skin layers are removed improving roughness, some discolorations, and fine lines.
Medium	Requires a few days of recovery time as some of the intermediate skin layers are removed, allowing the skin to regenerate with fewer fine and moderate wrinkles as well as discolorations.
Deep	Requires more than a week recovery time as the deep layers of skin are disrupted removing deeper wrinkles, acne scars, discolorations, and some precancerous growths.

Desired results from a chemical peel usually take several treatments. Optimally, superficial peels are performed every two to four weeks. The concentration of acid used may increase with each treatment as your skin becomes more tolerant. The total number of peels that you require will depend on your skin, the condition being treated, and which type of peel is used. Medium and deep peels often require just one treatment.

Microdermabrasion

Microdermabrasion involves the use of tiny firm crystals that are propelled toward and across the skin, and then removed by suction pressure. The movement of these particles against the skin causes small abrasions on the surface of the skin. As the skin heals, improvement in the quality of the epidermis and dermis occurs. Some instruments make

A microdermabrasion procedure takes approximately 20 minutes to perform, and there is minimal discomfort.

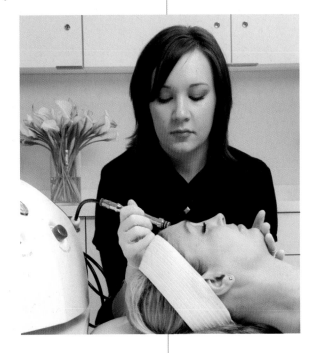

use of a diamond wand rather than loose crystals, but otherwise work in the same way. Microdermabrasion exerts its effects on different layers of the skin and can achieve different depths.

The depth is determined by several factors, including the type and size of the crystals used, the speed of the crystals, the amount of suction used, and by the technique of the operator, including the speed with which the wand is moved across the skin and the number of passes she takes. Depending on what is being treated and the skin type of the patient, microdermabrasion may include epidermal treatment, papillary dermal treatment, or reticular dermal treatment. It is similar to chemical peels in this way.

Microdermabrasion and chemical peels share other similarities. Like chemical peels, microdermabrasion is another form of superficial skin resurfacing. Also like chemical peels, microdermabrasion is used to treat conditions such as photodamage, acne, melasma, post-inflammatory hyperpigmentation, fine lines, and scars. It does tend to result in minimal erythema, and therefore has a short recovery time.

> Microdermabrasion will help a variety of skin problems including acne, fine lines, and skin discoloration.

How do you know whether a chemical peel or microdermabrasion is the right choice for you?

Both procedures are safe and effective for all skin types, and either may be a fine choice. Sometimes this decision is already made by your doctor because different doctors have a strong preference for one method or the other. Beyond that, the decision is an individual one that is best made in partnership with your doctor.

DIFFERENCES BETWEEN A CHEMICAL PEEL AND MICRODERMABRASION

Chemical Peel	Microdermabrasion
Chemical peels involve the application of an acid to the surface of the skin, to create a controlled destruction of the uppermost layers of the surface of the skin.	Microdermabrasion uses a stream of crystals or a diamond wand and suction to gently exfoliate the skin.
Chemical peels come in different strengths: superficial, medium, and deep.	Microdermabrasion's strength may be altered by changing the crystals, suction, or size of the wand used.
Deep chemical peels sometimes require an anesthetic.	Microdermabrasion does not require an anesthetic.
Deeper peels work well on superficial skin defects as well as more serious skin problems such as deep scars and wrinkles.	Works well on superficial skin defects such as fine lines and enlarged pores.

Botulinum toxin

The injection of botulism toxin (also known as Botox) has become one of the most widely used procedures in aesthetic medicine. The desire for improvement in appearance, reduction in lines and wrinkles, and the preference to avoid surgery when possible have all made botulinum toxin an extremely popular antiaging intervention. It is an effective treatment with a good safety profile and millions of satisfied users.

You probably know that botulism is a disease that is acquired by the ingestion of food contaminated with the bacteria *Clostridium botulinum* or by a wound becoming infected with the bacteria. The bacteria secrete a toxin that causes muscle paralysis and can be life threatening, especially if the respiratory muscles are affected. There are seven different forms of the toxin, labeled A through G. Fortunately, botulism is not an infection that occurs commonly.

Botulinum toxin injection for the removal of frown lines is the fastest growing cosmetic procedure in the United States.

There are times when doctors actually want to paralyze muscles in a very controlled way. For instance, there are people who have spasms of the eye or of the vocal chords. Diluted forms of botulinum toxin may be injected into these areas to temporarily eliminate the spasms. The eye conditions strabismus and blepharospasm and the voice condition spasmodic dysphonia are all effectively treated with the injection of botulinum toxin.

Very diluted concentrations of the botulism toxin can also be injected into the muscles of the face or neck in order to relax the muscles that cause wrinkles. It is particularly useful for frown lines, forehead wrinkles, and crow's feet. It is also used sometimes to relax the platysmal bands that give the neck a tense appearance.

In the United States there are two brands of botulinum toxin type A that have been approved by the FDA for cosmetic use. Botox was approved in 2002, and Dysport (formerly known as Reloxin) was approved in 2009. In 2001, Health Canada approved botulinum toxin type A for the treatment of frown lines. In the UK, Botox is also known as Vistabel. Botulinum toxin type B is also available to doctors. Brand names include Myobloc and Neurobloc. While botulinum toxin type B is not approved by the FDA, many doctors have significant experience with its use.

What should you expect at your treatment session? The doctor will first examine you and will ask you to make different faces in order to properly

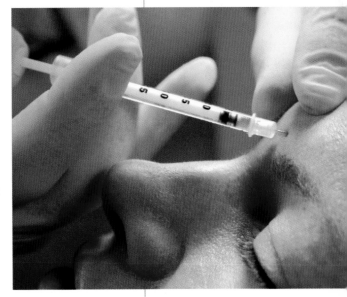

Injection of botulinum toxin into the corrugator supercilii muscles that cause frown lines relax the muscles cause and the lines to recede.

identify your musculature. You will receive a few or several injections depending on the treatment areas involved. The needle used is small, so most people comment that the discomfort is mild or moderate. The doctor may massage the injection site immediately after injection.

Dermal fillers

Dermal fillers are substances that are injected into the dermis in order to eliminate the appearance of medium and deep wrinkles and to augment the volume of the lips and cheeks. There are several different types of fillers available. Each offers advantages and disadvantages. Ultimately the decision of which filler to use will be made by your doctor. However, it is up to you to clearly articulate your desires and expectations in order to help him or her make a good choice. Some factors that go into the decision of which filler to use include the location and depth of the correction desired, the duration of time the correction should last, and the doctor's familiarity and comfort with individual products. In fact there are often several good options for filling any specific defect.

Collagen is the substance in the dermis that provides the skin's firmness, so collagen is often replaced in skin that has started to lose its support and develop wrinkles. The first injectable fillers were made from bovine (derived from cows) collagen. Because approximately 3 percent of the population is allergic to the bovine collagen, allergy testing is necessary before a patient can begin treatment. While several new products have been developed and are in use since the introduction of bovine collagen, it still remains in use because it is effective and it is less expensive than some of the newer agents. For most patients the results last between three and six months. Brand names for bovine collagen products include Zyderm I and II and Zyplast.

Because of the inconvenience of the allergy testing and because of the number of people allergic to the bovine collagen, the industry was sparked to develop a non-allergenic collagen product. Human collagen produced by fibroblasts from engineered skin is used in a similar fashion to the bovine collagen. It has the benefit of not requiring allergy testing and also lasts about 3 to 6 months. Cosmoderm I and II and Cosmoplast are frequently used.

More recently, a porcine (derived from pigs) collagen has been developed. It doesn't have the same level of allergenicity as bovine collagen, and so does not require allergy testing prior to use. Porcine collagen also has the added benefit

Cosmetic fillers are materials injected underneath the skin to fill in depressed or sunken areas.

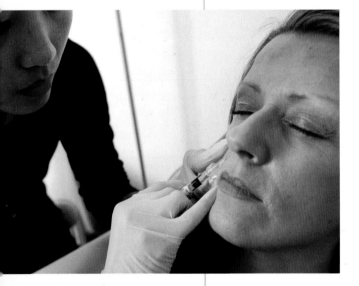

DERMAL FILLERS			
Filler (brand name)*	Source	How does it work?	Duration
Collagen (Cosmoderm, Cosmoplast, Evolence, Zyderm, Zyplast)	Derived from bovine, porcine, or human sources	Adds to the skin's natural collagen	3–12 months depending on type used
Hyaluyonic acid (Hylaform, Juvederm Ultra, Juvederm UltraPlus, Perlane, Restylane)	Derived from bacterial or avian sources	Boosts the skin's hyaluronic acid and then stimulates collagen production	3–12 months depending on type used
Calcium hydroxyapatite (Radiesse)	Synthetic calcium hydroxylapatite similar to the components of bone and teeth	Provides a scaffold upon which the skin can form new collagen	12–24 months
Poly-L-lactic acid (Sculptra)	Synthetic alpha hydroxy acid (AHA)	Boosts the skin's production of collagen; Stimulates the body to produce new collagen adding volume over time	24 months

*Also available in Canada

of lasting a bit longer than either bovine or human collagen—roughly 12 months. The brand name is Evolence.

Hyaluyonic acid is a substance that occurs naturally in the body. It is one of the more popular dermal fillers because it lasts longer than the collagen fillers do. Depending on which product is used and the location, these fillers can last 6–12 months. Of course every product has advantages and disadvantages, and the disadvantage of this product is that it can be more painful than the collagen injections. It also is more likely to cause bruising initially. Brand names include Restylane, Perlane, Juvederm, Prevelle, Puragen, and Captique, which are derived from bacteria, and Hylaform, which is derived from bird sources. It is important to note that different brands are available and approved in different countries.

SKIN SOLUTION

Calcium hydroxylapatite is the primary component of bone and teeth. Synthetic calcium hydroxylapatite (such as Radiesse) can be used as a dermal filler to provide a scaffold upon which the skin can form new collagen.

Calcium hydroxyapatite filler is also known by the brand name Radiesse. It contains calcium hydroxyapetite particles in a polysaccharide gel. The gel gets absorbed by the skin, and the particles are left behind in the upper dermis where the doctor places it. Those remaining calcium hydroxyapetite particles likely act as a scaffolding around which the body forms new collagen. The results of this filler may last 12 months or more. It is particularly useful for the nasolabial folds, marionette lines, cheeks, chin, and temporal wasting. Due to the risk of cyst formation, use for lip augmentation is not advisable.

Poly-L-lactic acid is a volume enhancer, unlike the other products that are true fillers. In the United States it was first FDA approved for the treatment of HIV lipoatrophy, and now it is approved for improving facial wrinkles and sunken areas of the face.

SKIN SOLUTION

There are many different types of lasers, and new ones are developed each year. Lasers can help to improve a variety of problems such as excessive hair growth, birthmarks, brown or red discoloration, and deep wrinkles. Remember, laser treatments may not be right for everyone as special precautions must be taken with darker skin tones.

Lasers and other devices

Lasers have vastly improved the number of medical and cosmetic treatment options available to patients. In essence, lasers emit a focused beam of intense light that has a very specific target in the skin, causing little surrounding tissue damage. They have the ability to treat many skin conditions effectively. However, it is important to see a trained doctor because lasers can also have unwanted side effects, including permanent scarring, if used without caution, without proper training, or on the wrong skin type.

There are many dermatologic uses for lasers. They can be used to remove unwanted hair; to treat skin discoloration from melasma, the

LASERS FOR COSMETIC USE	
Used to remove	**Common laser types**
Wrinkles	Carbon dioxide Erbium YAG
Hair	Long pulse Nd: YAG Diode
Scars	Carbon dioxide Erbium YAG Fractional carbon dioxide
Discolorations	Q-switched YAG Q-switched alexandrite
Blood vessels	Pulsed Dye KTP
Tattoos	Ruby Alexandrite

sun, and postinflammatory hyperpigmentation; to smooth the texture of the skin and tighten it; to treat vascular lesions such as broken blood vessels and some birthmarks; to remove tattoos; and to treat photodamage and remove precancerous lesions. With so many useful applications, it is no wonder that laser centers have become so common.

There are several different types of lasers available and dozens of brands. One condition may be treatable by several different lasers. A doctor's choice of laser will depend on your skin type, the condition to be treated, and what lasers she has at her disposal.

Sclerotherapy

Unsightly leg veins can cause you to want to wear pants or long skirts all of the time. Sclerotherapy is a procedure during which your leg veins are injected with a solution that will make the veins disappear. It is preferred to surgery because it is less invasive with faster healing. Although lasers have been used to treat leg veins, they are most successful with the tiny varicose veins or the small squiggly spider veins.

If you have larger leg veins, it is important to have an ultrasound or Doppler examination of your leg veins to see if the small superficial vessels that will be treated are connected with the deeper veins in your leg. This is because with sclerotherapy, after injection of the sclerosing liquid or solution, the blood ceases to course through the veins and a blood clot forms. The vessel is then absorbed over the next few weeks by the body. We do not want a blood clot to form in the deep veins of the legs (a serious condition called deep venous thrombosis). The ultrasound or Doppler procedure will ensure that a deeper connection does not exist.

When you undergo the procedure, a sclerosing solution is injected into the leg veins with a small needle. You may experience a small pinch from the needle and cramping of the muscles of the leg is possible. The procedure may take 20 to 40 minutes. Following the injections, the legs are wrapped with Ace bandages to provide compression that will collapse the small vessels.

After the first sclerotherapy session, you will see an improvement in the leg vessels, but often two or more treatments are required to achieve the desired result. The second treatment will likely be performed one month after the first treatment.

A foam sclerosant may be used, particularly for larger varicose

COMMON SCLEROSING AGENTS

- **Sodium tetradecyl sulfate**
- **Polidocanol**
- **Hypertonic saline**

WHAT YOU NEED TO DO BEFORE SCLEROTHERAPY

- **Avoid aspirin, ibuprofen, or other nonsteroidal anti-inflammatory drugs that can cause excessive bleeding.**
- **Do not apply lotion or creams to the skin prior to the procedure .**
- **Bring Ace bandages or compression stockings to wear after the procedure.**

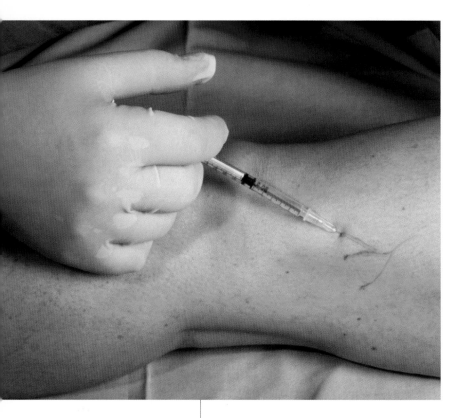

veins. This procedure is performed under ultrasound guidance to ensure that the foam is placed in the correct area.

There are potential side effects or complications associated with sclerotherapy. Allergic reactions to the sclerosing agent can rarely occur. A blood clot in the deep blood vessels, known as deep venous thrombosis, is a rare complication. Ulceration or necrosis of the skin overlying the blood vessel, and a brown streak where the blood vessel was originally located, may occur.

It is important to note that you are not eligible for sclerotherapy if you are pregnant or breast-feeding. However, you are permitted to have sclerotherapy if you take birth control pills.

A sclerosant is injected into a patient's leg to treat varicose veins. The paths of the veins are marked in purple on the skin.

At-home procedures

There are times when you may be unable to splurge and have a cosmetic procedure performed by a professional but you would still like to look better and improve your skin. Two common procedures that can be done at home are home-microdermabrasion and home-chemical peels. The first question that you should ask is what are the advantages, disadvantages, and risks of the at-home procedures? The overwhelming advantages are the lower cost and the convenience in terms of time and travel. The disadvantages are that you will have a lower strength of the active ingredients or a simulation of the actual procedure which means that your results will be

Before performing any at-home procedure, read all of the instructions on the box and follow them exactly as written.

more modest. You may also need to use the at-home variety more often to achieve your desired results. Since you are not a trained professional, you will also run the risk of side effects such as redness, discoloration, or bruising. To avoid these side effects, it is important that you follow the directions exactly as outlined on the box.

At-home microdermabrasion

At-home microdermabrasion kits usually contain creams with rough or abrasive particles that remove the very superficial layer of the skin. With some kits you will have to apply the cream with your fingers, while others will supply an applicator to apply the cream. The rough or abrasive particles will remove your dead skin cells, leaving the skin softer and smoother. The particles may be aluminum, magnesium, or even fruit seeds or pits. A moisturizing cream or lotion may be supplied in the kit as a final step.

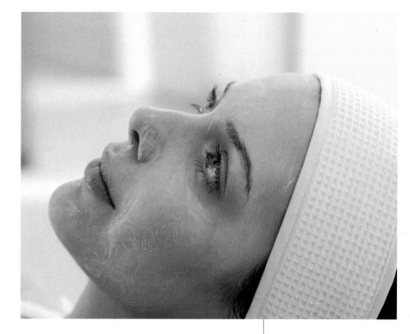

Even though the results will probably be slower, it is still possible to experience side effects such as redness, irritation, stinging, tingling, or burning. If any of these occur, discontinue use of the kit immediately.

At-home chemical peels

Similar to at-home microdermabrasions kits, at-home chemical-peel kits are designed to remove the most superficial layer of dead skin cells. Instead of using an abrasive agent, a chemical is used. The chemical will vary depending upon the kit, but often salicylic, lactic, malic, or glycolic acid may be the active ingredient. Sometimes papain derived from papaya is used.

Remember that acids have the potential of irritating or burning the skin so directions must be followed as outlined in the instructions. This in-home procedure will produce smoother, softer, and more even skin.

Cosmetic surgery

As the years pass, a number of factors lead to changes in how we look. These changes include heredity, sun exposure, smoking, alcohol, estrogen replacement, and the pull of gravity. Having a cosmetic procedure to reverse or minimize these changes may lift your spirits, improve your confidence, and give you a much needed boost to face the world. But don't think that cosmetic surgery will magically make the parts of your body that you do not like disappear. And don't imagine that you will be transformed into sheer perfection.

Never purchase or use a "professional"-strength chemical-peel product for use at home. Never leave the peel on longer than the directions indicate.

Skin Myth

True or False?
Cosmetic surgery will change your life.

False

It is important to have realistic expectations about your procedure. The decision to have cosmetic surgery should not be made lightly.

There are several principles that we encourage you to follow if you are considering cosmetic surgery. It is important that your doctor explain all possible side effects to you prior to the surgery. If you do not understand something, it is important that you ask as many questions as you need until you are satisfied and fully understand.

Finding the right doctor

Doctors of many specialties perform cosmetic procedures. It is up to you to investigate if the doctor that you have selected is qualified to perform your surgery. One assurance is if your doctor is board certified. Look for a board certified plastic surgeon, ophthalmologist, otorhinolaringologist (ear, nose, and throat doctor), or dermatologist depending on the procedure.

Other certifications may not assure you someone is well trained. Additionally, ask the doctor if he or she specializes in, and has extensive experience in, performing the procedure that you are considering. It is also valuable to get a second opinion from another doctor. Don't look for someone who is simply going to tell you what you want to hear. Ask to see before and after photographs of patients that the doctor has performed surgery on. Also, this is not the time to look for "bargain-basement" prices. Remember the saying, "you get what you pay for." For most procedures, you will be required to cover the cost of the surgical suite or procedure room, the anesthesiologist, the surgeon, and implant if there is one. Remember, there are side effects associated with all surgical procedures. It is important that your doctor explain all possible side

> Cosmetic surgery should never be taken lightly. It should be fully investigated and carefully considered before a decision is made.

PREPARING FOR SURGERY

Risks of surgery

All major surgeries have risks and the possibility of side effects, including:

- Bleeding
- Infection
- Scarring
- Pain
- Numbness
- Anesthesia reactions
- Serious complications, which can be fatal

Steps you can take to prepare for surgery

- If you're a smoker, you should stop smoking completely at least four to six weeks before your surgery.
- Do not diet before surgery since proper nutrition and well-balanced meals are important for the healing process.
- Your doctor may recommend taking certain vitamins such as vitamin A to assist with healing.
- Avoid medications that may cause excessive bleeding such as aspirin, ibuprofen, naproxyn, or other medications.
- Avoid vitamins and herbs that can cause excessive bleeding such as vitamin E and St. John's Wort.

effects to you prior to the surgery. If you do not understand something, it is important that you ask questions.

Anesthesia

Several factors help to determine what type of anesthesia you will have during your procedure, including the type of procedure, your physician's judgement and your preferences. Local anesthesia, which only numbs the area that will be worked on, is an option for some procedures. Other procedures will require general anesthesia where you will be totally unconscious and may have a breathing tube during the procedure. Sedation, where you are asleep but not totally unconscious, is a third option. Your doctor will ultimately make this decision with your input. It is important that you find out if what you want to physically achieve is indeed achievable with plastic surgery.

You must be realistic about what you want done and what the outcome will be. You also need to be prepared physically and emotionally for your procedure. Do you need to stop smoking or stop visiting a tanning salon to prepare your body for the surgery? Do you need to improve your intake of vitamins and other nutrients so that your body will heal properly?

Common cosmetic procedures

In the next few pages, we will discuss six of the most popular cosmetic procedures that are performed throughout the world:

1. Liposuction (lipoplasty)
2. Eyelid surgery (blepharoplasty)
3. Breast enlargement (augmentation mammaplasty) and breast lift (mastopexy)
4. Facelift (rhytidectomy)
5. Tummy tuck (abdominoplasty)
6. Nose surgery (rhinoplasty)

In addition, gastric bypass will be discussed since it is a serious surgical intervention for obesity, and has dramatic effects on one's appearance.

Liposuction

Have you noticed a layer of fat around your tummy or bulging hips, buttocks, or thighs? Have you tried exercising and your fat pads just won't budge? If the answer is yes, then liposuction may be for you. With

In general, liposuction is a well tolerated surgical procedure. Immediately following the procedure, you may experience some soreness, bruising, and swelling, but you should bounce back quickly.

During liposuction fat is removed with a hollow tube called a cannula, through which the fatty deposits are extracted with either a syringe, or a suction pump.

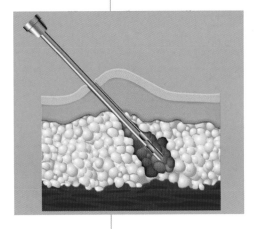

this procedure, the excess fat is removed or "sucked out." But it is important to realize that liposuction will not cause you to lose weight. Instead it will help to shape and contour the area that is treated and remove your bulges. If you are overweight, liposuction is not for you. Instead, you should exercise and modify your eating before you have liposuction. Although liposuction actually removes the fat cells beneath the surface of the skin, it does not remove or improve cellulite. The effects of liposuction will last a long time assuming that you do not gain weight after the procedure. The best results occur in people with good skin elasticity so that the skin will not sag or appear loose after the fat is removed. There are several ways that liposuction can be performed.

Tumescent liposuction is the most common technique. With this form of liposuction, a small hole is made in the skin, a saline solution is injected into the area, and the fat is removed with a small tube called a cannula. The fluid helps the doctor remove the fat. The cannula is attached to a vacuum that sucks the fat and fluid from beneath the skin's surface.

Ultrasound-assisted liposuction is the next technique, and a metal rod that sends out sound waves is inserted beneath the surface of the skin. The sound waves break up the fat and turn it to liquid, which allows it to be removed more easily. Although skin burns can occur, it works very well for people who have thick, dense fat cells.

After fatty deposits are removed with liposuction, your abdomen will be noticeably flatter and your waist streamlined.

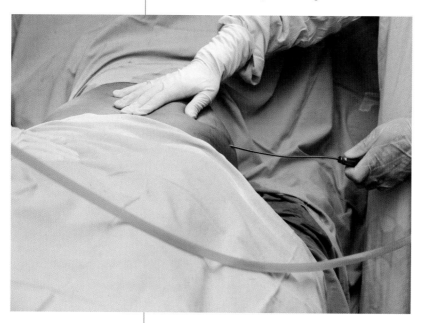

Powered liposuction is the final technique that is commonly used. With this technique, the cannula moves in a very fast back-and-forth motion, which produces vibrations. The vibration allows thick, dense fat to be removed more easily. This technique is also used in small areas, such as the knee or ankle area because of its precision.

Complications that may occur with liposuction are: a bumpy or wavy appearance of the skin; numbness in the area treated; discolorations of the skin; pockets of fluid; infection; internal organ punctures; and death. These complications are rare, and there are treatments that can minimize or treat the side effects.

Pain, swelling, bruising, and small irregular lumps of fat occur commonly after the procedure. You will be instructed to wear a tight compression garment to help reduce swelling for a few weeks. The fat irregularities will disappear as the remaining fat settles into position. It takes about four weeks for most of the swelling to subside. After six months, the area treated will appear lean and tight. After your procedure, always inform your doctor if anything seems abnormal.

Eyelid surgery (blepharoplasty)

If you are sick of people asking you whether you are tired or did not get enough sleep because of the bags under your eyes, then eyelid surgery may be for you. Also, if you have sagging of your upper eyelids or extra skin that is starting to block your vision, then you, too, should investigate eyelid surgery. As many people reach about 50 years of age, the muscles that support the eyelids weaken and the eyelids stretch. This causes drooping of the upper lids, sagging of the eyebrows, and the appearance of dark bags under the eyes. Eyelid surgery, which we call blepharoplasty, or "bleph" for short, removes the excessive droopy lid skin and the fat pads that cause the bags, and it tightens the muscles. However, a "bleph" will not improve crow's feet, droopy eyebrows, scowl lines, or hoods that droop down from the outer corner of the eyelids. There are other procedures that can help those problems. Crow's feet and scowl lines can disappear after an injection of botulinum toxin. Eyebrows and droopy eye hoods may be lifted during a facelift procedure. Blephs may be performed

The dotted lines above and below the eye show where incisions will be made to remove excess fat, along with skin and muscle.

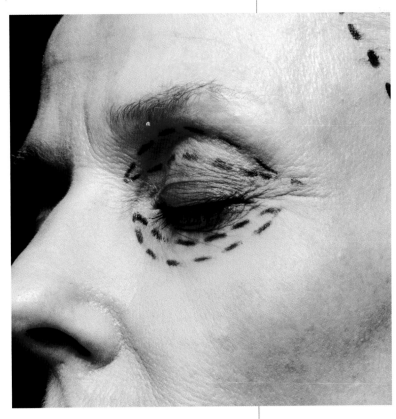

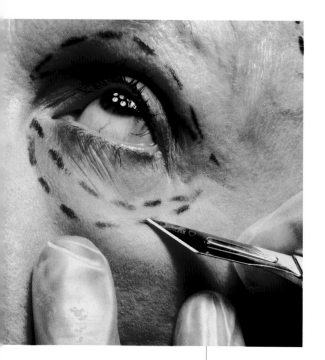

A blepharoplasty can be performed quickly, with most procedures completed in an hour.

by a board certified ophthalmologist, plastic surgeon, or cosmetic dermatologist under local anesthesia with mild sedation that will make you groggy. During the procedure, the upper eyelid skin is cut along the crease of the eye; the excess skin and muscle is removed with a scalpel; and the skin is closed with very small stitches that leave a nearly invisible scar. For the lower lid, a cut is made just below the eyelashes or on the inside of the lower lid. The surgeon removes excess fat pad, sagging skin, and muscle. Then small stitches are placed to close the incision. If the incision is made on the inside of your eyelid (on the pink conjunctiva), you will not have a scar at all on your skin, but your eyes may be more swollen after the surgery.

After the surgery you may expect swelling, discoloration, a "black eye" or numbness for a few days to a week. Potential side effects associated with a "bleph" include: temporary numbness of the eyelid skin; dry, irritated eyes; eyelids that do not move properly; scarring; and a small risk of blindness.

Breast enlargement (augmentation mammaplasty) and lifting sagging breasts (mastopexy)

Breast enlargement, also called augmentation mammaplasty, is a procedure that enlarges the breast by inserting implants below the breast tissue or below the chest muscle. The procedure is performed for women who are

SILICONE VS. SALINE IMPLANTS		
Type of implant	**Advantages**	**Disadvantages**
Silicone	• More natural looking • Lower rate of rippling and wrinkling • Very light so lower risk of downward displacement as a result of gravity	• More expensive than saline • Longer scar • Higher risk of capsular contracture • May rupture "silently," leaving no outward evidence
Saline	• Lower rate of revision surgery • Lower risk of capsular contractures • Less expensive than silicone • Smaller scar • If the implant ruptures, the saline is absorbed into the body	• May look round and feel stiff and unnatural • Heavier than silicone so more likely to succumb to gravity

not satisfied with their breast size, or for women born with one breast larger than the other. This surgery may be performed under local anesthesia with sedation or general anesthesia. During the surgery, the implants are inserted through an incision that your doctor makes either in the crease under your breast, around the nipple, or in your armpit. There are two types of implants: silicone and saline. It is important to discuss the advantages and disadvantages of each type with your doctor. After the incision is made, the surgeon inserts the implant into a pocket created either in front of or behind the chest muscle.

It is important to be realistic about the size of your implants and your new breasts. You probably do not want implants that are out of proportion with your body frame or your overall size.

There are several things that you must know and discuss with your surgeon before your surgery. Breast implants don't last forever. It is likely that they will need to be removed and replaced at some point. A study of saline implants determined that as many as 25 percent of women required a second operation within five years of the insertion of their implants. If your implants are removed, you may have dimpling, drooping, or wrinkling of the skin that will require additional surgery to fix these problems. You also have to consider the size of the scar created by the surgery.

There is the possibility that your implants could rupture or break and the fluid could leak into the breast and surrounding tissue. The implants will lose their size or shape (deflation) and your doctor may order an MRI (magnetic resonance image) to check if a rupture has occurred. It is also important to know that breast implants will not prevent your breasts from sagging or improve sagging if you already have it. If your breasts sag, you will need a breast lift (mastopexy).

After breast augmentation you might experience changes in the sensation of your breasts. If your incision is made around your nipples it may affect their sensation as well. Also, you may feel the implant beneath the surface of the breast tissue. Breast augmentation can make breast-feeding difficult or impossible and mammograms may be more difficult for the radiology doctor to interpret.

During breast augmentation surgery, the initial incision may be placed along the circumference of the areola. The surgery may affect the nerves of the skin and produce altered or decreased sensation.

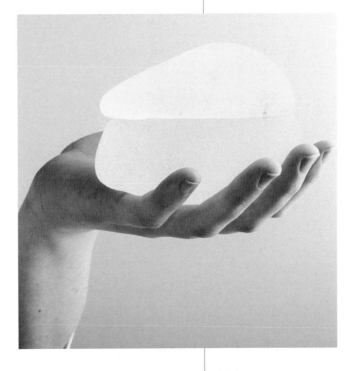

There are additional side effects that can occur shortly after surgery. These include infection, hematoma (collection of blood or fluid), and pain. Antibiotics are usually effective in treating the infection, but there have been instances where removal of the implant has been necessary for cure.

Hematomas may cause pain, infection, or other problems. If you develop a hematoma, you might need to go back into the operating room so that your doctor can find the cause of the bleeding, stop it, and remove the excess fluid. After surgery, it is possible for scar tissue to form and create a capsule around the breast implant. The capsule will constrict the implant, a condition called capsular contracture. The scar tissue may be painful and disfiguring but can be corrected with surgery.

You should have realistic expectations regarding your surgery and appearance afterward. Understanding the size, shape, and feel of your breasts after the implant is very important to having an outcome that you are satisfied with.

> Since it will take about two weeks for complete healing of a facelift with resolution of swelling and bruising, you should plan to miss work and social activities during that period of time.

Facelift (rhytidectomy)

Many women entering their 50s and 60s notice that their facial skin becomes loose and the nasolabial folds, the area between the corner of the nose and mouth, become prominent. Crow's feet develop at the corners of the eyes. Forehead lines form deep folds and frown lines appear. Jowls form along the jawline, and a double chin may develop. The area under the cheekbone may become hollow. For many women, when they look in the mirror, their facial appearance does not match the way that they feel or think of themselves.

Almost all of those unwelcomed changes can be significantly improved with a facelift (rhytidectomy). There are factors that help to determine the success of your final results, such as the elasticity of your skin, your ability to heal,

During a rhytidectomy, the surgeon will make an incision around your ear as demonstrated here before excess tissue is removed.

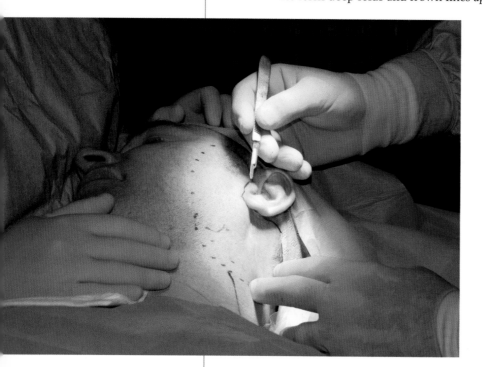

your bone structure, skin type, ethnic background, and your expectations. It is important to know that having a facelift will not stop the aging process.

For the procedure, which usually takes two to four hours, either local anesthesia with sedation or general anesthesia may be used. There are several different ways in which a facelift may be performed. In general, your surgeon will make an incision in front of and behind the ear and up into the scalp. The skin is raised outward, muscles are tightened, and fat and excessive skin are removed. Small stitches or metal staples are used to close the incision. A drainage tube may be inserted during surgery that will be removed one or two days after surgery. A bandage may be wrapped around your face. Elevation of the head is extremely helpful in reducing the swelling. The stitches will be removed five to ten days after surgery.

The most common side effects are swelling, bruising, and discoloration. Additionally, infection, hematoma (an accumulation of blood under the skin), numbness, and reactions to anesthesia may occur. Scars may develop as a result of surgery, but they are usually well hidden by positioning them in the natural skin creases and in the hairline.

Assuming that you limit sun exposure, do not smoke, and take care of your skin, you may expect the results of your facelift to last six to ten years. In general, your surgeon will probably perform another facelift if you desire another one at that time.

Tummy tuck (abdominoplasty)

If you are tired of doing sit-ups with no results and the flab on your abdomen won't budge, then you might want to consider a tummy tuck (abdominoplasty). Pregnancy, dramatic weight changes, gravity, and aging can all lead to sagging of the abdomen. A tummy tuck will flatten your abdomen by removing extra fat and skin and tightening the abdominal wall muscles. You are a good candidate if you are not planning more pregnancies, and you are at your ideal weight.

The tummy tuck procedure can take between one and five hours

PROBLEM AREAS HELPED BY FACIAL SURGERY
Crow's feet
Forehead lines
Double chin
Sagging eyelids

ARE YOU A GOOD CANDIDATE FOR ABDOMINOPLASTY?	
Reason	**Yes/No**
You have loose tissue after pregnancy (and are not planning any more pregnancies).	Yes
You have sagging skin after weight loss and are now at your ideal weight.	Yes
You would like a tighter, flatter stomach.	Yes
You would like this to be a treatment for weight control.	No
You want to substitute surgery for regular physical activity and a healthy, balanced diet.	No

During an abdominoplasty, although the incision is made at the bikini line, excess fat, muscle, and skin are removed from most of the abdomen and muscles are tightened.

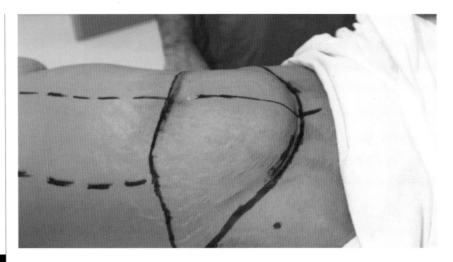

to complete, and it is performed under general anesthesia. There are several techniques that your doctor can choose from to perform your surgery. The first procedure is called a complete abdominoplasty. It involves cutting the abdomen from one hip all the way across to the other hip. The incision is made at the level of the pubic hair so that it can be camouflaged if you wear a bikini. Then the skin, fat, and muscles are removed and rearranged. Your belly button will be repositioned. Drainage tubes may be placed under your skin for a few days.

Mini-abdominoplasty, or a partial-abdominoplasty, is the second type of tummy tuck procedure. This procedure is appropriate for people whose fat deposits are located below the navel and need only a short incision. Fat, skin, and muscle will be removed and rearranged. The belly button will probably not be repositioned during this procedure.

There are several expected side effects associated with your tummy tuck that include pain, swelling, bruising, and scarring at the incision site. Numbness of the skin may occur, and you may feel tired after the procedure. Other complications may include infection and bleeding: these are rare but have been reported.

Rhinoplasty
Many people are not happy with the appearance of their nose. Some people feel that their nose is too large, too long, too pointy, too bumpy, or too wide. A rhinoplasty is a surgical procedure that can correct the problem with your nose. In fact, rhinoplasty is a popular procedure for people of all races and ethnicities. Often individuals of East Asian decent will request a rhinopolasty to narrow the shape of the nose and raise the nasal bridge. Individuals of African descent often request narrowing of the nostrils.

Individuals of Caucasian descent often request removal of the hump near the bridge of the nose. Although rhinoplasty is most commonly performed for cosmetic purposes, it is also performed for a variety of medical conditions.

Although the nose is a small structure, it consists of several layers including the underlying bone and the flexible cartilage, which are covered by fat and skin. Inside the nose is a structure called the septum that divides the right from the left side of the nose. There are two ways that a rhinoplasty can be performed, either a closed or an open approach. With closed rhinoplasty, several incisions are made inside the nose, and with the open procedure, in addition to incisions inside the nose, another is made across the segment of the skin that connects the nostrils, called the columella. With these procedures, after the skin and underlying tissues are reflected back, the cartilage and bones are reshaped. Bone and cartilage may be removed or extra pieces of cartilage or bone may be added to change the shape of the nose. The incisions are then repaired with stitches. The nose is packed inside, and tape or a plaster cast is applied.

Side effects or complications may occur, as with all procedures. Bleeding and infection are potential problems. Numbness of the tip of the nose lasting several months is not uncommon. Scar tissue can form inside the nose, causing breathing difficulty, which could require additional surgery to remove. The septum inside of the nose can be inadvertently punctured forming a hole, called septal perforation, which would require repair.

It has been estimated that the results of between 5 percent and 20 percent of rhinoplastys are unsatisfactory to the patient. This can occur if too much bone or cartilage is removed, and the nose will appear deformed and assume the shape of a beak or alternatively will flatten across the bridge producing the appearance of a saddle. Variations in the surgical technique

Profile of a woman's face before and after undergoing cosmetic surgery to reduce the size of her nose.

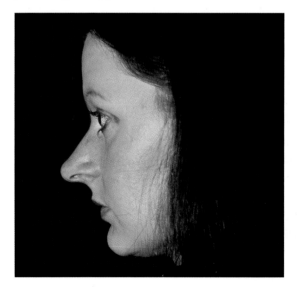

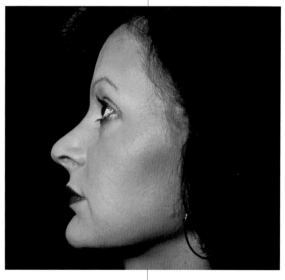

- Nasal destruction due to trauma from an accident
- A collapsed nose from perforation of the nasal septum
- Correction of nasal obstruction following a previous cosmetic surgery
- Skin cancer removal
- Enlargement of the nose from rosacea (rhinophyma)
- Nasal deformity from birth
- Improvement in the appearance of the nose

could produce side effects that may include a nose with nostrils that are too visible, or nostrils that have a pinched look. If you do not like the result or look of your rhinoplasty, a secondary rhinoplasty, also called a revision rhinoplasty, can be performed. Also, if there is a problem such as the growth of excess tissue that interferes with breathing, a revision rhinoplasty may be performed to correct this.

Finally, depending upon the problem that you would like corrected, a non-invasive and non-surgical rhinoplasty may be performed using a filler substance. Common fillers include Restylane, Juvaderm, Evolence, and Radiesse, which are injected through a needle. If, for example, there is a depression on the nose you would like to minimize, it can be filled in with one of the filler substances. A hump on the bridge of the nose can be minimized or smoothed by injecting a filler around the hump. Since surgery is avoided, so too are many of the potential complications. Redness, bruising and swelling may occur immediately after the injections but resolves rapidly. It is important to know that use of fillers in this way, although often performed by physicians, is not approved by the FDA in the United States.

Gastric bypass

Gastric bypass is used as a treatment for obesity and its related illnesses. It

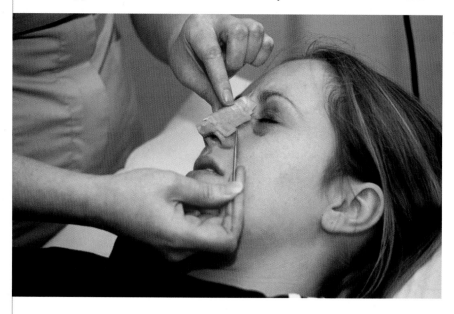

A nurse removing a plaster from the nose of a woman one week after a rhinoplasty operation. The bruising around the patient's eye developed after her nose was broken during the surgery.

can cause a significant change in your overall appearance. So, when you think that losing 100 pounds or more to attain your ideal weight is an impossible task, you may wish to consider gastric bypass surgery. The principle behind gastric bypass is to reduce the size of your stomach so that you will not be able to eat as much food as before the surgery and your body will not absorb all the calories from the food you eat.

Today, instead of your surgeon using a large incision to open your abdomen and expose your stomach for the gastric bypass, a laparoscope is used. This small flexible tube has a camera on the end that allows your surgeon to view your stomach on a video monitor in the operating room. Using the laparoscope and very small instruments, your stomach size can be reduced after making only a very small incision.

As you can imagine, laparoscopic surgery is preferred for several reasons:

- Less invasive than open surgery
- Requires only 4 to 6 small incisions
- Leads to faster healing for the patient
- Results in smaller scars
- Lower risk of developing a hernia

In addition to inserting the laparoscope through one of the incisions, thin surgical instruments are inserted through the other small incisions, and a gas such as CO_2 is injected to allow enough room for the surgeon to work and manipulate the instruments.

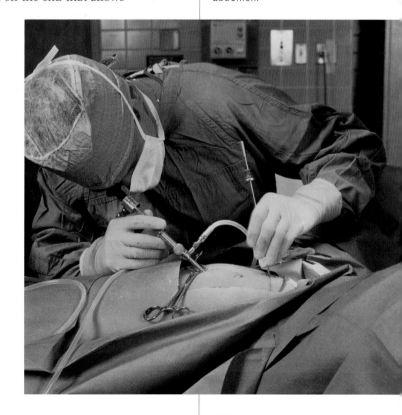

A surgeon using a laparoscope to examine the inside of a patient's abdomen.

You may wonder exactly how the surgeon bypasses the stomach. First, staples are used to divide your stomach into a small pouch about the size of a walnut, and into a larger section at the bottom. You will not feel the staples because the surgery is performed under general anesthesia, which means that you will be asleep during the surgery. The second step involves bypassing the larger section of the stomach by attaching a part of the small intestine called the jejunum directly to the small pouch. With this procedure, food bypasses the lower part of the stomach as well as the first part of the small intestine, called the duodenum.

At the completion of the surgery, your new stomach will only hold approximately 1 ounce (30 g) of food, and you will absorb fewer calories. If you overeat after your surgery, your new small stomach will be unable to hold the food and you will vomit.

Gastric bypass surgery may be suitable if you are obese and have not been able to lose weight with diet and exercise.

Serious risks and side effects can occur, as with all surgical procedures. It is important that you understand and discuss these risks fully with your surgeon before you commit to your surgery. Possible side effects are varied. They may be related to anesthesia, rapid weight loss, or the new stomach size and re-routing of the intestine. Side effects sometimes reported after surgical procedures like the gastric bypass include bleeding or infection, blood clots in the legs, irregular heartbeat or heart attack, stroke, or even death.

Examples of stomach and intestine side effects include injury to the stomach, intestines, or other organs during surgery. Breakdown of your small stomach pouch could occur, which would necessitate surgical repair. The lining of your stomach may become inflamed producing heartburn or ulcers. The opening from the pouch to the intestine could become too small for food to pass through and another surgery would be necessary. The food in your stomach could move through your intestine too quickly, a condition called

A laparoscopic adjustable gastric band is used to shrink the functional size of the stomach.

dumping syndrome, causing discomfort and poor nutrition. Improper absorption of nutrients from food may occur, leading to poor nutrition, which could result in anemia and weakness or even thinning of the bones due to low calcium absorption. Rapid weight loss can result in gallstone formation with resulting pain.

After surgery, people lose about half of their weight after two years, with approximately 10 to 20 pounds (4.5 to 9 kg) lost each month. The weight loss does not just happen. It requires discipline, hard work, exercise, and a special diet.

Laparoscopic adjustable gastric band is a newer procedure, also know as Lapband, that has been developed. It achieves the same goal as gastric bypass, reducing the size of the stomach. This procedure involves the placement of a silicone band around the upper part of your stomach to reduce its size. There are several advantages to the Lap-Band procedure as compared to standard bypass surgery, and it is now the preferred procedure for many people contemplating weight-loss surgery.

Following surgery, extra care must be taken, particularly relating to eating and drinking so as not to place a strain on the stomach pouch, which could cause the Lap-Band to slip out of place. Immediately after surgery and for a few weeks, it is important to consume only liquids, graduating to pureed foods. This will allow the stomach to heal properly. Examples of pureed foods include pureed skinless chicken or fish, mashed potatoes, peas, low-fat yogurt, or pudding.

An amazing aspect of the Lap-Band is that it can be adjusted based upon your pouch size, the amount of weight that you wish to lose, and the rapidity with which you desire to lose weight.

LIQUIDS RECOMMENDED AFTER LAP-BAND SURGERY

- Water
- Clear broth or soup
- Skim milk
- Fruit juice
- Sugar-free popsicles

Nutritional counseling prior to your surgery is very important to learn what and how much to eat.

ADVANTAGES OF LAP-BAND PROCEDURE

- Minimally invasive
- Often does not require hospitalization
- Faster healing and return to activities
- Intestine not re-routed, avoiding "dumping" syndrome
- Stomach not stapled, obviating those side effects
- Procedure reversible with stomach returning to its original shape

5

Skin and Your Health

Your skin is just like any other organ in your body; taking care of yourself helps it to function optimally and can help you look your best. What does this mean for you? Eat a diet rich in fresh fruits, vegetables, legumes, and whole grains. These foods are nutrient rich and contain antioxidants that help fight the free radicals that contribute to aging.

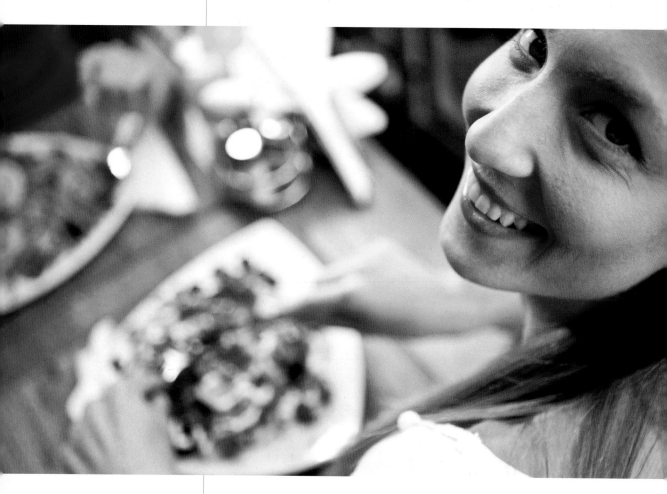

Your overall health

A balanced diet is essential for good overall health. It is the foundation for a healthy body. Beyond that, your doctor may suggest that you take a multiple vitamin, as well as fish oil for cardiovascular protection, and vitamin D and calcium to ensure good bone health. Adequate hydration with water, as opposed to soft drinks or juice, is also important for overall good health.

The sun and your health

The sun enables us to produce vitamin D, which is important for strong bones and for our immune and endocrine systems to function properly. Vitamin D is also available through food sources, including fish such as salmon, mackerel, and tuna and in fortified foods such as milk. Vitamin D deficiency is a very common problem. Numerous studies have documented a high prevalence of vitamin D deficiency in children, adolescents, and adults. While the prevalence rates reported vary from study to study, some researchers have documented vitamin D deficiency rates of over 80 percent. People of all ages are at risk, and in the United States the problem is more prevalent for African-American women than for Caucasian women. The sun emits radiation that is characterized by its wavelength which can be helpful in treating certain diseases. The light that actually reaches the Earth includes ultraviolet C, ultraviolet B, ultraviolet A, and visible light. Light therapy has been proven effective in treating certain skin conditions, see the box below.

Types of skin cancer

According to the American Cancer Society, skin cancers including basal cell carcinoma, squamous cell carcinoma, and melanoma account for more than half of all cancers in the United States. Therefore it is vital that you perform a monthly self-examination (see chapter 1) and visit your dermatologist for regular checkups.

Basal cell carcinoma

Basal cell carcinoma (BCC) is the most common of all cancers, affecting

---

LIGHT TREATMENTS

Light treatment, also termed phototherapy, utilizes the power of ultraviolet light to treat certain skin disorders. Your doctor may refer you to phototherapy if you have psoriasis, eczema, vitiligo, or intractable itching. Some doctors treat seasonal affective disorder (SAD) with light as well.

The most common types of light treatments are: Psoralen and ultraviolet A light (PUVA), broadband ultraviolet B (UVB), and narrowband ultraviolet B (nbUVB).

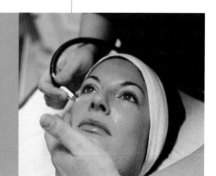

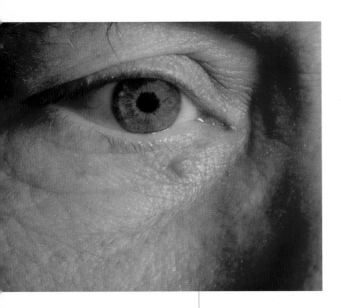

The classic appearance of basal cell carcinoma is a pink, pearly papule with a slight depression in the center.

approximately 800,000–900,000 people in the United States annually. Basal cell carcinomas arise from the cells of the basal layer of the skin that sit at the base of the epidermis. They can occur anywhere on the body, but they occur most often in sun-exposed areas. This includes the face, ears, chest, back, hands, and forearms. They may also occur in scars and the sites of previous irradiation.

Basal cells are easily recognizable but have a few different appearances. Sometimes they are translucent papules, meaning that they are small bumps that have a "see through" appearance. You can sometimes see small blood vessels within them. Sometimes BCCs look like pimples or sores that won't heal. If you have a spot that bleeds on and off and never goes away, you should have it evaluated. Sometimes BCCs look like shiny pink spots, and sometimes they have pigment in them and are brown rather than flesh colored.

Fortunately, BCCs tend to be very slow-growing. While they are much less likely to metastasize than some other skin cancers, they can grow quite large and can be quite destructive locally, at their original site. A BCC can go beneath the skin to destroy the cartilage of the ear or nose, or to expose the muscle underlying the skin in other areas of the body. For this reason it is important that you don't just ignore a spot that you think might be a basal cell carcinoma.

Basal cells can be treated in a number of different ways. How your physician decides to treat your BCC will depend on its size, location on your body, and on the form of BCC you have. Some types are more aggressive than others. The physician may elect to do a simple excision, where the skin around the basal cell is cut out in the shape of an ellipse, and then the skin edges are stitched back together. Sometimes a doctor will decide to do an electrodessication and cautery (ED&C). In this procedure, the basal cell carcinoma is scraped with a curette and burned with an electric needle. This cycle is repeated, usually three times.

Moh's surgery is named after a general surgeon, Dr. Frederic E. Mohs. It is used to treat many types of skin cancers, and reduces the likelihood of recurrence.

For BCCs on the face or with aggressive pathology, you may be referred to a Moh's surgeon. With the Moh's procedure, the smallest amount of skin necessary is taken, while ensuring that all the cancer has been removed. The surgeon looks at the sample under the microscope while you wait to ensure that the edges of the sample are free of tumor.

Squamous cell carcinoma

Squamous cell carcinoma (SCC) is the
second most common skin cancer, affecting
approximately 200,000–300,000 people in the
United States annually. These tumors arise from
the keratinocytes higher up in the epidermis.
They are usually pink patches or plaques and may
be a little scaly. They are often on sun-exposed
areas but may also occur in sun-protected areas.
SCCs commonly occur in scars, burns, and
other sites of previous trauma. They may also
arise from actinic keratoses, the gritty-feeling,
rough red spots that come from too much sun exposure. People who are
immunosuppressed are more likely to develop SCCs. Also, exposure
to human papilloma virus (HPV) increases the risk of SCC. SCCs can
metastasize. For this reason, it is important to treat them early. SCCs are
usually treated by excision, or, in certain cases, by Moh's surgery.

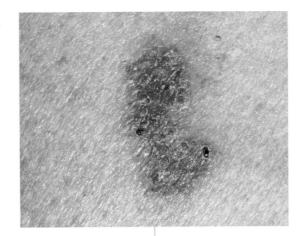

Squamous cell carcinoma
in situ, also called
Bowen's disease, only
involves the epidermis
and may appear as a red,
scaly patch on the skin.

You may be told that you have an SCC in situ. This condition is also
called Bowen's disease. This means that the cells look cancerous, but they
have not gone below the level of the epidermis. This means that it has been
caught early.

Melanoma

While melanoma is less common than BCC or SCC, it is responsible for the
majority of skin cancer deaths. It arises from melanocytes in the epidermis.

The incidence of melanoma is rising around the world and in different
ethnic groups. When caught early, melanoma has a 99 percent 5-year
survival rate. Unfortunately, when melanoma is not caught early, and has
spread it has a 18 percent 5-year survival rate. This means that it is very
important to educate yourself about melanoma so
that you know what to look for and know when
it's time to go to the doctor.

The characteristic
appearance of
malignant melanoma:
an asymmetric, irregular
border; dark color; larger
diameter growth on
the skin.

Remember that everyone is at risk for
developing melanoma. Some people do have an
increased risk, though. How can you tell if you
are at increased risk? There are two simple tasks
that you can do to decide. First, talk to your
relatives. Having a family history of two or more
relatives with melanoma means that you are
genetically more susceptible to it as well. Second,
look in the mirror. If you are fair-skinned, if
you have a large number of nevi (moles), or if
you have atypical-appearing nevi, then you are

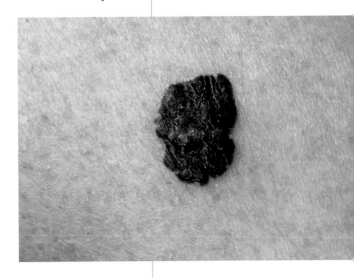

at increased risk for developing melanoma. While everyone should have a full-body skin exam performed by a dermatologist every year, people at increased risk for melanoma should be particularly diligent.

Skin self-examination

As previously discussed in chapter 1, in addition to annual skin exams, you should perform a skin self-examination monthly. This allows you to become familiar with your skin and to rapidly identify any new growths or changing lesions. In order to perform a self-examination properly, you will need a large mirror as well as a hand mirror so you can see all areas of your body. You will look for growths that look unusual and take note of the ABCDE's (asymmetry, border, color, diameter, evolution). In addition, you should pay close attention to lesions that continually scab or bleed and those that do not heal within three weeks. If during your self-examination you see a spot that raises concern, or if you are just not sure about a specific lesion, then you should see your dermatologist immediately. Don't just wait for your next annual skin check. Remember that with melanoma, early diagnosis is the key to survival.

What next?

If your doctor suspects melanoma, what should you expect at your visit? Your doctor will take a thorough history, including a family history, if she has not done so already. You will have an examination that will likely include looking at your skin and feeling your lymph nodes, liver, and spleen. Depending on the size and location of the lesion and her level of suspicion, your doctor will make a decision about what type of biopsy is best. She may recommend an excisional biopsy, where the whole spot is cut out and your skin is stitched back together. Or she may perform a saucerization where the whole spot is scooped out but no stitches are necessary. Alternatively, a punch biopsy may be performed, removing the entire lesion if it is small. Finally, while it is less common, in some cases a doctor will choose to do a partial biopsy.

If you are diagnosed with melanoma, then what? You will receive a further workup, which will be guided by the depth and other characteristics of the tumor itself, the information that you give your doctor concerning your general health, and your physical exam. While their value is still debated by physicians, your doctor may recommend a sentinel lymph node biopsy. The

Cutaneous T-cell lymphoma can appear as a flat or raised rash, or very occasionally with tumors on the skin.

OTHER TYPES OF SKIN CANCER

- Cutaneous T-cell lymphoma
- Cutaneous B-cell lymphoma
- Merkel cell tumor
- Cutaneous metasteses of tumors from other organs

sentinel lymph node is the first lymph node where cancer cells may spread from the primary tumor. If your tumor is deep or if distant spread is suspected, you may also have imaging studies such as an MRI of the brain; a CT scan of the chest, abdomen and pelvis; or even a whole-body PET scan. Ultimately, you will be given a stage that reflects the depth of the tumor, whether or not there are lymph nodes involved, and whether or not the cancer has spread to other parts of your body. Your stage will provide you information about your prognosis.

Skin cancer prevention

Like many things in life, it's much simpler to prevent skin cancer than it is to treat it. By preventing skin cancer, you will not face the risks of surgery, you will avoid the scar that comes from removing a cancer, and you will prevent the risks of local destruction and distant spread that a skin cancer carries with it. Prevention also saves time going to the doctor for skin cancer treatments and the associated costs.

Skin cancer prevention practices are very easy, especially those related to sun exposure. Protection involves shielding the skin from the sun, either with the use of sunscreen, protective clothing, or both. Skin screenings are necessary to identify precancerous and cancerous lesions as early as possible.

Risk assessment

How do you know how much sun protection you need? The UV index is a good guide. It is a prediction of the amount of ultraviolet radiation that will be present the next day. The index value is correlated to your risk of

SKIN SOLUTION

If a skin biopsy is recommended by your dermatologist, there is no reason to worry. The procedure will take less than 5 minutes and you will receive numbing medications so the procedure will not hurt.

The vast majority of sun damage occurs before age 18 so it is very important to protect your children from sun exposure throughout their childhood.

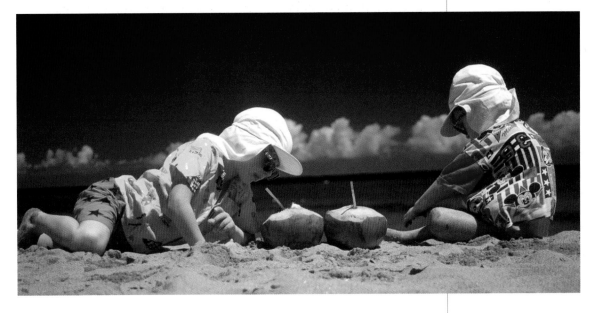

overexposure to the sun, ranging from "low" to "extreme." When the amount of UV radiation is predicted to be unseasonably high in an area, the EPA issues a UV alert. Knowing the UV index lets you estimate how much sun protection you will need in a given day.

Sunscreen

It is important to look for sunscreen with UVA and UVB protection, and at least SPF 30 in most cases. Sunscreen needs to be reapplied every two hours, and after you get out of the water. Sunscreens are discussed extensively in chapter 2.

Protective clothing

There are several companies that manufacture sun protective clothing. These clothes are intended to provide a barrier between the skin and harmful ultraviolet rays. This clothing may work in different ways. A fabric may be effective based on the density of its weave, based on the dyes contained in the fabric, or because it has been pre-treated with ingredients that provide protection by absorbing UV light. Protective clothing typically covers the body well: for example shirts are long-sleeved, hats have a wide brim, and shorts and skirts are often long as well.

> Clothing is very important in protecting your skin from the sun, but only if it is tightly woven or pretreated with ultraviolet light absorbers.

Protective clothing may be rated with a UPF designation. This stands for Ultraviolet Protection Factor, and it is a measure of how well an item protects against UVA and UVB. Some clothing just reports its SPF, which is only an indication of UVB protection.

UV protection is also an important consideration when choosing eyewear. UV light can harm the eyes, causing macular degeneration, which is damage to the retina that can lead to blindness. It also seems to lead to a greater risk of cataracts and other problems. Don't assume that just because sunglasses are tinted that they are providing protection. Lenses must be specially coated with a UV protectant, unless the lenses are made of polycarbonate. If you are unsure about whether or not your lenses are providing UV protection, you should check with your optometrist.

THE IMPORTANCE OF SUN SAFETY

Sun safety is a lifelong commitment. It must begin in childhood and continue throughout life. You will likely get most of your sun damage before you are 18 years old. Daily use of sunscreen, wearing sun protective clothing and hats, and seeking shade are all important habits to have.

Early detection

Everyone should have an annual skin cancer screening by a professional. If you have already had a skin cancer, or if you are at an increased risk, your physician may want to see you even more frequently. This exam should include all of your skin and mucous membranes. It is important that you arrive at the doctor's office prepared for this exam. You should use minimal hairspray and few hairclips or ponytail holders so that the doctor can part your hair to examine your scalp easily. You should also avoid wearing nail polish on your fingers or toes so that the nail beds can be examined. You should expect the doctor to look inside your mouth, as well as examine areas like the genitals and rectum. Because skin cancer can occur anywhere, it is important that all of these areas be checked. If you have numerous moles or unusual looking moles, then your physician may opt to photograph them.

Tanning salons

There are many different reasons that people go to tanning salons. Some people enjoy the way their skin looks when it is tan. Some people like the feeling of the light on the skin. Others think that if they get a "base" tan before going to the beach they are actually protecting their skin. None of these are good justifications for going to a tanning salon.

Unfortunately, tanning beds are just not safe for the skin. They emit primarily UVA and a smaller amount of UVB light in order to provide the skin with a tan. These beds accelerate the skin's aging process, and they significantly increase the risk of basal cell carcinoma, squamous cell carcinoma, and melanoma. In one study, women who tanned at the salon once a month were 55 percent more likely to develop a melanoma later in life.

The appearance of tanned skin can be achieved safely using a variety of cosmetic products. Bronzers and self-tanners are discussed in detail in chapter 2. Self-tanners can be applied at home or can be obtained from a salon where the use of an airbrush machine provides a particularly even and natural-looking application.

It is important to note that occasionally people with medical conditions are treated with ultraviolet light. Diseases like eczema, psoriasis, and chronic itch are often controlled with light treatments. Please remember that treating a disease under a physician's supervision is not the same as going to the tanning salon for cosmetic reasons. And, even light treatments under physician supervision carry risks that should be discussed with your doctor before beginning treatment.

You should never go to a tanning salon. The ultraviolet light in the tanning bed may harm your skin, producing skin cancer, premature aging, and even eye damage.

Skin Myth

True or False?
There have been reports of young women in their 20s, who used tanning beds, developing melanoma skin cancer.

True

Hormones and your skin

Think of hormones as chemical messengers that circulate throughout your bloodstream. Estrogen is one such hormone, and it directs a woman's body to develop in the characteristically female ways. There are three stages of life when our bodies undergo great changes because of dramatic differences in this hormone. Puberty, pregnancy, and menopause are each influenced by estrogen: production begins in puberty; surges of estrogen occur during pregnancy; and dramatic decreases in estrogen occur during menopause. With each stage, there are significant differences in a woman's skin and hair.

Puberty

In North America and Europe, puberty begins between the ages of 8 and 14. It is characterized by changes in hormone levels. When estrogen levels increase, there are many changes in a girl's skin. Puberty signals the onset of hair growth on the body, body odor, and acne. Hair begins to grow in the pubic area, under the arms, and on the legs. The hair is dark in color and may be coarse, curly, or straight. Body odor begins during puberty and is strongest in the underarm area and in the genital area.

Your menstrual cycle is a complex 28-day cycle in which key hormones, including estrogen and progesterone, cause shedding of the lining of the uterus.

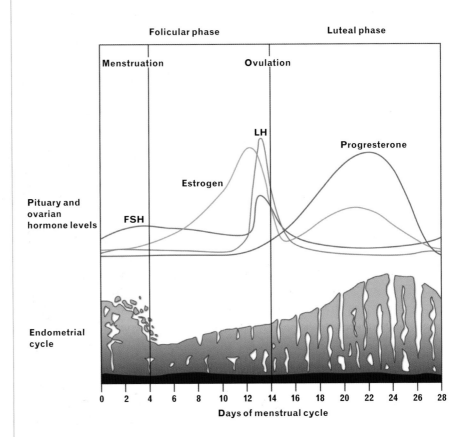

Acne is a problem for many young people. It begins during puberty and is directly related to the stimulation of oil glands by hormones. A combination of excessive oil, bacterial growth, and plugging of pores leads to blackheads, whiteheads, and pimples on the face, chest, and back. Despite what many teens may think, acne is not caused by dirt. Treatment targets oil, bacteria, pores, and inflammation. It is fine to begin treatment with over-the-counter products containing either benzoyl peroxide, salicylic acid, or sulfur. If these medications do not result in an improvement in the acne after six to eight weeks of use, then a pediatrician may prescribe medications such as tretinoin, adapalene, or tazarotene, which are effective in unplugging the pores. Additionally, either topical or oral antibiotics can help control the bacteria responsible for acne. If hormonal levels are abnormal, oral contraceptive pills may regulate the hormone levels.

It is important to caution teens not to wash vigorously or more than twice a day. Over-washing and scrubbing the skin can lead to significant irritation. Teens also tend to over-use medication by applying too much (only a pea-size dot is needed to cover the entire face) or applying it more often than instructed by their doctor.

SKIN SOLUTION

Acne first appears at the onset of puberty when androgen hormones in the body stimulate skin cells to produce oil. The oil is then used by the skin's bacteria as fuel and they proliferate. Additionally, pores become plugged or blocked. Treatment is directed at decreasing the bacteria, reducing oil, and unplugging pores.

During pregnancy many changes occur in the skin, such as the appearance of the linea nigra, a dark line extending from the chest bone to the pubic bone.

Pregnancy

The hormones released during pregnancy can play havoc with your skin and outward appearance.

Skin tags may occur during pregnancy. These benign growths are extra pieces of skin that may hang off of the neck, the underarm area, or under the breasts. Since they are harmless, they do not need to be removed unless they become uncomfortable.

Moles may change during pregnancy and become somewhat larger in size or darker in color. It is important to show any changing mole to your doctor just to make sure that it is nothing to worry about. Typically, the moles will return to normal after delivery.

Acne may worsen during pregancy.

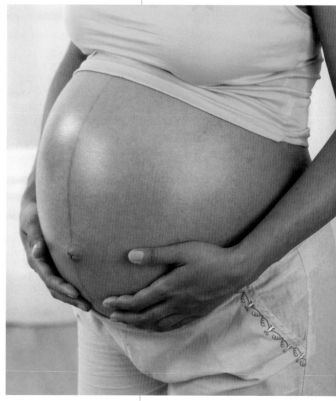

Skin color changes, particularly the darkening of certain areas of the body, are common during pregnancy. On the abdomen, a brown line stretching from below the chest bone to the pubic bone, the linea nigra, becomes prominent. The areolae surrounding the nipples become darker as does the genital area. These skin discolorations fade after delivery. Melasma, commonly referred to as the mask of pregnancy, is a skin discoloration affecting the face. Dark patches appear on the cheeks, upper lip, and forehead. Sunlight worsens the condition. Melasma may not disappear after delivery and has been known to last for years afterward.

Blood vessel growth is often pronounced during pregnancy. Small red blood vessels that look like spiders (spider angiomas) may grow on the face, neck, and arms. Unlike the larger varicose veins on the legs, spider angiomas frequently resolve after delivery. Varicose veins, however, usually require a surgical procedure for resolution.

Hair and nail changes occur during pregnancy. Many women report long, thick hair on their scalp throughout their pregnancy. However, hair loss can occur approximately three months after delivery, a condition called telogen effluvium. Hair with white balls on the end is a hallmark of telogen effluvium. Telogen effluvium may last for six months or longer with subsequent regrowth of all of the hair. Many pregnant women have accelerated growth of their nails during pregnancy. However, nails may become brittle and grooves may appear on them. This usually resolves after delivery.

Menopause

The onset of menopause occurs when estrogen levels in a woman's body decrease. Smooth, moist skin may suddenly become dry and thin. Moisture may be replaced with a variety of moisturizers that will need to be applied daily. Thinning of the skin means that not only are superficial blood vessels more easily seen, but bruising also occurs more easily. Taking extra care to avoid even minor injury to the skin will minimize bruising. Benign growths appear on the skin with the onset of menopause, such as the warty or crusty growths referred to as seborrheic keratosis, which seem to multiply at this time in life. Since they have no cancerous potential, these growths do not have to be removed. If they bother you, they can be frozen, burned, or cut off by your dermatologist. Skin tags are another benign growth that seem to multiply during menopause. They commonly appear as skin-colored growths that hang off of the skin especially on the neck, underarms, and under the breasts. They can be easily removed.

SKIN SOLUTION

Performing a skin self-examination monthly is important to ensuring that pre-cancerous and cancerous growths are identified early. Simply check your skin from head to toe. Use a mirror to look at your back, buttocks, backs of your legs and difficult to see areas. Don't forget to look at your hands, feet, nails and between your toes.

Androgenic alopecia is a type of hair loss that is more likely to affect women who enter menopause. With this type of hair loss, there is thinning in the crown area of the scalp that may move forward toward the hairline. Fortunately, topical minoxidil (Rogaine) may be helpful in slowing down the hair loss, and it may stimulate some regrowth. Additionally, loss of hair may also occur in other areas of the body. Thinning of the eyebrows as well as loss under the arms and in the pubic area may be seen.

Hair changes are seen all over the body. Just as distressing as the hair loss is the growth of unwanted hair, particularly on the chin. Eflornithine cream (Vaniqa) may be helpful in slowing down hair growth. Laser hair removal may also be helpful as long as the facial hairs have not turned gray. Speaking of gray hairs, they begin to appear even faster after menopause begins. Various hair dyes or rinses are sufficient to cover gray hair.

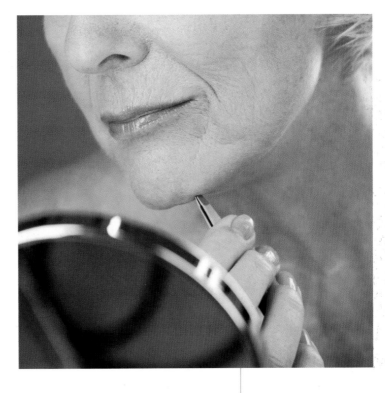

Excessive hair growth, termed hypertrichosis, often occurs on or under the chin. Effective treatments are available.

Medications and your skin

Medications that you take for a variety of reasons, from those that control your blood pressure or your diabetes, to those that control seizures or those that prevent pregnancy, can all have an effect on the appearance of your skin.

Side effects of medication

Some medications can cause an increased sensitivity to the sun with redness, burning, or darkening of the skin. Others can cause hair loss on the scalp or excessive hair growth elsewhere. There are medications that can cause or worsen common skin problems such as acne or cause something as common as dry skin. Some of these possible adverse side effects are listed in the table on the following page. If you are worried about the possible side effects of your medication, speak to a professional.

Never use your friend's or family member's acne medication. Everyone's skin is different, and the wrong medication may in fact harm your skin.

MEDICATIONS WITH POSSIBLE ADVERSE SIDE EFFECTS

Can increase sensitivity to the sun

- Acne medications: Adapalene (Differin), Tazarotene (Tazorac), Tretinoin (Retin A)
- Antibiotics: Doxycycline, Minocycline, Tetracycline
- Antiseizure medications: Phenytoin (Dilantin)
- Birth control pills
- Blood pressure: calcium channel blockers (Diltiazem), Hydrochlorothiazide

Can cause hair loss

- Antidepressants: Amitriptyline (Elavil), Lithium, Fluoxetine (Prozac), Tri-cyclics
- Antiseizure medications: Valproic acid
- Birth control pills
- Blood pressure: beta blockers, Atenolol (Tenormin)
- Blood thinners: Warfarin (Coumadin)
- Vitamins: Vitamin A in high doses

Can cause excess hair growth

- Antibiotic: Streptomycin
- Antihypertensives: Diazoxide
- Antirejection medications for transplants: Cyclosporin
- Antiseizure medications: Phenytoin (Dilantin)
- Glaucoma medication: Acetazolamine

Can cause dry skin

- Acne medications: Isotretinoin (Accutane)
- Antidepressants: Paroxetine (Paxil), Fluoxetine (Prozac), Sertraline (Zoloft)
- Cholesterol-lowering drugs: Atorvastatin (Lipitor), Ezetimibe and Simvastatin (Vytorin)
- Lupus medications: Hydroxychloroquine (Plaquinel)
- Psoriasis medications: Acitretin (Soriatane)

Can cause or worsen acne

- Antidepressants: Lithium
- Antiseizure medications: Phenytoin (Dilantin)
- Antituberculosis medications: Isoniazid, Rifampin
- Anabolic androgenic steroids: Danocrine (Danazol), Stanozolol (Stomba)
- Birth control medications: Medroxyprogesterine (Depo-Provera)
- Corticosteroids: Dexamethasone, Methylprednisone, Prednisolone, Prednisone
- Thyroid medications: Propylthiouracil

The skin: A window to your body

Your doctor more often than not thinks of your skin as the window to your body. By simply looking at your skin, he or she can tell if your circulation is poor or if you have diabetes or even if you are pregnant. How is this possible? There are signs that may appear on your skin or on your hair and nails that can reveal the inner workings of your body. There are signs that signal good health such as pink nail beds. On the other hand, there are signs that may indicate a problem such as a crease or line on your earlobe. In this section, we will discuss signs that you should know about that serve as a window into your body's health.

Cardiovascular system

The cardiovascular system consists of your heart, which pumps blood throughout your body, and blood vessels that carry your blood. If there is a blockage in a blood vessel, you will not have enough blood flowing to that area of your body. This condition is referred to as poor circulation. For example, if the blockage occurs in your legs, this means that the tissues of your legs, including the skin, will not get enough oxygen or nutrients. A lack of oxygen affects the skin color of the legs and toenails, and both may become blue or gray. There may also be a loss of hair on the legs. If your doctor sees abnormal skin color and sparse or missing hair, he or she will suspect poor circulation and order tests to evaluate your blood vessels.

A blockage in the artery that supplies blood to the heart will cause a heart attack (myocardial infarction). There is a sign that can be found on your earlobe that can tell you about the condition of your heart. A diagonal crease on your earlobe can be a sign of heart disease. This has been demonstrated in several different studies. Some believe that the crease can signal to your doctor that you may be at risk for a heart attack.

High levels of cholesterol can block your arteries and lead to heart attacks. These elevated levels can cause yellow spots on or near your upper eyelids. The spots, called xantholasma, are actually deposits of cholesterol and related lipids. They are a signal that your cholesterol and lipid levels should be checked. If your levels are elevated, you should change your diet and possibly begin cholesterol-lowering medication.

A clear artery will supply all of the required blood to the part of the body that it supplies. Plaque buildup in an artery will cause a partial or complete blockage that will reduce the flow of blood.

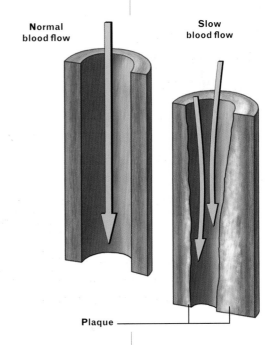

Normal blood flow

Slow blood flow

Plaque

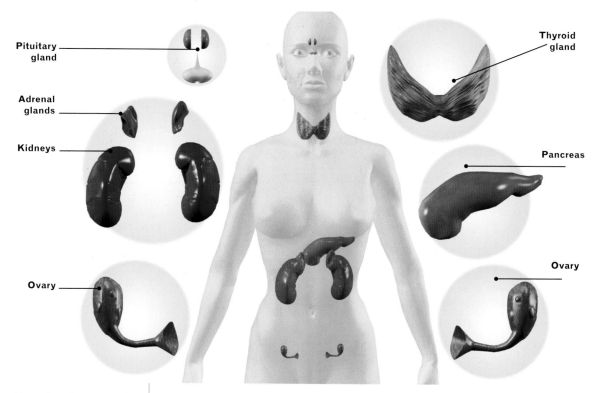

Pituitary gland

Adrenal glands

Kidneys

Ovary

Thyroid gland

Pancreas

Ovary

Examples of components of the endocrine system are the pancreas that produces insulin, the adrenal gland that produces cortisone, and the thyroid gland, that produces thyroid hormone.

The endocrine system regulates vital body functions such as height, weight, growth, metabolism, sexual development, and fertility.

Endocrine system

The endocrine system is very complex and encompasses several organs as well as the hormones that they produce. The thyroid gland, pancreas, testicles, and ovaries are a few of the organs that make up the endocrine system of your body. The organs of the endocrine system make and secrete hormones that allow your body to function properly. For example, the pancreas secretes the hormone insulin, which controls your blood sugar level. If your pancreas does not make enough insulin, your blood sugar levels will rise, and you will develop diabetes mellitus. It would be very helpful if your doctor could see an early sign of diabetes on your skin, even before ordering a blood test. There are two signs that may occur on your skin that indeed signal diabetes. Likewise, there are signs that may appear on your skin that signal a problem with your thyroid gland or even your ovaries. Simply read on to learn what to look for.

Diabetes

Dark, velvety patches on the back and sides of your neck that are sometimes mistaken for dirt but do not wash away may be an early sign of diabetes. In Type 2 diabetes, the pancreas initially secretes large amounts of insulin, but the body is resistant to the insulin. The dark patches on the neck, called acanthosis nigricans, appear because high levels of insulin in the body stimulate the skin cells to produce extra cells that are dark in color. Patches may also develop under the arms, on the face, and chest.

Raised brown patches on the shins of your legs may also signal diabetes mellitus. These patches, called diabetic dermopathy, are usually the size of a pack of cards and may resolve with treatment. Diabetic dermopathy is reported to occur in up to 40 percent of individuals with diabetes.

Hyperthyroidism and hypothyroidism

Signs of an overactive or underactive thyroid gland may be seen in changes in both your skin and hair. Either can cause hair loss on the scalp. With a hyperactive thyroid, your skin may become warm and moist. With hypothyroidism, hair loss can occur along the outer edge of the eyebrows. The skin and scalp may be cool and dry.

Polycystic ovarian disease

Guess which organ is not functioning properly if a woman has a combination of facial acne pimples, hair loss on the scalp, and excessive hair growth in the beard area. An abnormality of the ovaries of women, polycystic ovarian disease, is responsible for this constellation of changes. With polycystic ovarian disease, the ovaries do not develop or function properly and the normal amounts of the hormone estrogen are not made. Women with this disorder find that their acne does not improve with medication, that they develop facial hair, and experience thinning hair on the scalp.

SKIN SOLUTION

Diabetic dermopathy lesions appear most frequently on the shins and are harmless. They usually do not require any treatment and tend to go away after a few years, particularly following improved blood glucose control.

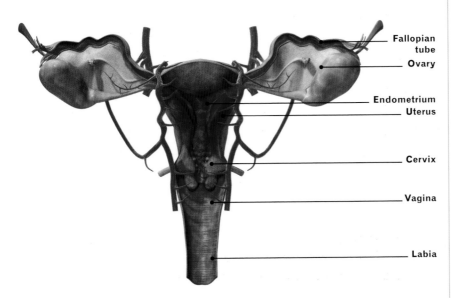

Fallopian tube
Ovary
Endometrium
Uterus
Cervix
Vagina
Labia

The female reproductive system.

Pregnancy

Changes in skin color on the face, breasts, and abdomen may signal pregnancy. Dark patches on the cheeks, upper lip, chin, and forehead can also signal that you are pregnant. This skin disorder, melasma, may occur in women all over the world. Unfortunately, it does not always resolve after the birth of the baby. Other skin-color changes that occur during pregnancy are a darkening of the skin on the breasts and a dark line stretching from the belly button down to the pubic bone and worsening of acne.

Pulmonary system

Problems with our lungs affect our ability to breathe properly. These very lung problems can also be reflected in our nails. When nails become yellow in color, also known as yellow nail syndrome, this signals that the body is not receiving enough oxygen.

SKIN SOLUTION

Since sunlight is known to exacerbate lupus, it is critically important to protect your skin from the sun if you suspect you have lupus. Your doctor can order a blood test or perform a skin biopsy to determine if you do indeed have this disorder.

Immune system

Our body's immune system helps us fight infection, and it protects us from substances that our bodies consider foreign. If the immune system malfunctions or goes into hyperdrive, several diseases may develop. Lupus is just one such disease, and it can produce several different types of rashes on the body. The most commonly known rash associated with lupus is the so-called butterfly rash. This red facial rash is shaped like a butterfly. Hair loss on the scalp and red blood vessels around the fingernails can also be important signs of lupus.

Good nutrition: A recipe for healthy skin

We all know that good nutrition is a recipe for healthy bodies and skin, and many countries have a national food guide to help their citizens meet their essential vitamin, mineral, and nutrient requirements. China, Philippines, Singapore, Indonesia, Thailand, Malaysia, Vietnam, Canada and the United States each have guides. Most nations recognize four food groups: vegetables and fruits, grain products, dairy and dairy equivalents, and protein in the form meat and its alternatives.

A good example of a national food guide is the United States Department of Agriculture Daily Food Guide. It allows you to have an idea of the foods that you will need each day. Also remember that the types of protein, fruits, vegetables and carbohydrates will vary depending on where you live. In the United States and Canada bread, cereals, and pasta are popular carbohydrates that serve as the base of the food pyramid. In Asia corn, rice, legumes, seed, and nuts provide the foundation for the diet. Meat and

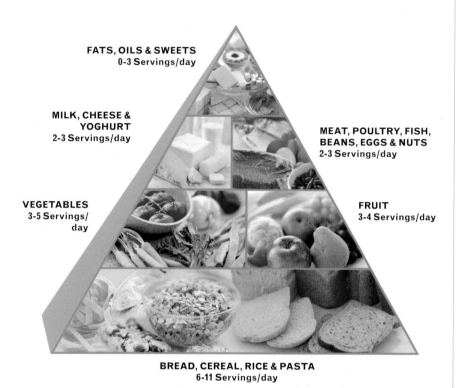

FOOD PYRAMID

FATS, OILS & SWEETS
0-3 Servings/day

MILK, CHEESE & YOGHURT
2-3 Servings/day

MEAT, POULTRY, FISH, BEANS, EGGS & NUTS
2-3 Servings/day

VEGETABLES
3-5 Servings/day

FRUIT
3-4 Servings/day

BREAD, CEREAL, RICE & PASTA
6-11 Servings/day

poultry are the forms of protein most often consumed in North America whereas tofu, fish, and shellfish are proteins consumed most in Asia.

U.S. Department of Agriculture's Daily Food Guide

The food pyramid is a handy guide to show you how to eat a healthy and balanced diet every day. This is not a strict guide and obviously every person has different needs, depending on a wide range of factors such as age, sex, weight, and height.

Carbohydrates

The foods at the base or the bottom of the pyramid are the ones that you should eat the most of, but it is important to note the size of the portions that are recommended. Six to eleven servings of three ounces (85 g) of whole-grain bread, cereal, rice, crackers, or pasta are recommended each day. This means no "super-size" servings. Additionally, it is important to minimize sugar and high-glycemic carbohydrates including potatoes, white rice, and pasta that can cause blood sugar to spike and create free radicals

Skin Myth

True or False?
Carbohydrates are an important component of your diet and should not be eliminated.

True

Although it is important to eliminate sugary and processed foods from your diet, whole-grain carbohydrates such as bread, pasta and cereal are important for a healthy diet.

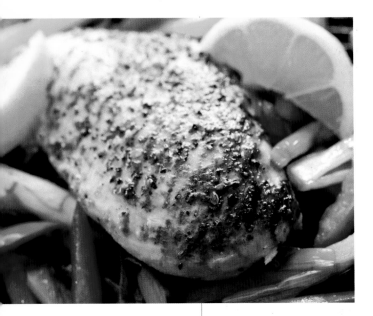

(that are harmful to your skin). However, your body does need carbohydrates so select and eat low-glycemic fruits and vegetables.

Fruits and vegetables

Two to four servings of fruits and three to five servings of vegetables are recommended daily. Remember to include dark green and orange colored vegetables in your diet, since these will provide your body with the most nutrients.

Protein

The higher up on the pyramid a food is, the less you should consume of it. Protein-rich meats, poultry, and fish should be eaten less often than fruits, vegetables, and other healthy carbohydrates. Although these foods are important in cellular repair, selecting the correct type of protein-rich foods is important. So, for example, you want to select low-fat or lean meats. For poultry, remove the skin on the chicken or turkey, which removes much of the fat. Fish is always a good choice, but some types are actually high in cholesterol, such as shrimp, or high in fat, like salmon, and so consumption should be moderate.

Poultry is a good source of protein, but don't forget to remove the skin because it contains fat.

Dairy

Dairy is an important source of calcium that is responsible for strong bones and the health of your teeth. Calcium is particularly important for women during puberty, pregnancy, and menopause. The daily intake requirements increase during those periods of life. Milk, cheese, yoghurt, and fish bones (sardines, mackerel) are great sources of calcium. Select fat-free or low-fat milk and other dairy products.

SKIN SOLUTION

Antioxidants are highly recommended for healthy skin because they trap potentially harmful free radicals. Free radicals may damage skin cells and lead to precancerous and cancerous growths.

Fats and oils

Everyone needs some fat in their diet. It helps absorb some vitamins and helps you to feel full. Some fats actually protect against heart diesease, improve brain health and may protect against cancers. Look for fish that contain omega-3 fatty acids such as salmon, mackerel, and albacore tuna. Also, extra-virgin olive oil and flaxseed oil provide the right types of fat for your diet.

Antioxidants

We have mentioned several foods that are rich in antioxidants. It is important to understand why it is vital to have a diet rich in antioxidants. Free radicals are generated by ultraviolet light, smoking, pollution, and normal cellular functions. Free radicals produce inflammation that damages skin cells, leading to skin cancers and premature aging. Antioxidants act as free radical scavengers to prevent or reduce inflammation and subsequent damage to your skin cells. The skin's antioxidant reservoir is derived primarily from foods. Dietary antioxidants include vitamin C (ascorbic acid) and vitamin E (tocopherol).

Vitamins and your skin

So you might wonder how vitamins C and E can directly help your skin. A recent study demonstrated that the skin of individuals who ingested vitamins C and E for three months had less sunburn when exposed to the ultraviolet B burning rays of the sun. Also, there was less damage to the cell's DNA after ultraviolet B radiation, which indicates that these two vitamins can protect against DNA damage. Other vitamins, such as vitamin A, have been found to maintain and repair skin tissue. The B vitamin, biotin, is responsible for forming the basis of skin, hair, and nail cells.

> For women of all skin types, supplements are the best way to ensure adequate Vitamin D levels.

FOODS HIGH IN VITAMINS C, D, AND E		
Vitamin C	Broccoli Citrus fruits Green peppers	Strawberries Sweet and white potatoes Tomatoes
Vitamin D	Cod liver oil, 1 tbsp. Egg, 1 whole (egg yolk) Liver, beef, cooked, 3 oz. (85 g) Mackerel, cooked, 3 oz. (85 g) Margarine, fortified, 1 tbsp. Milk, vitamin D fortified, 1 cup	Ready-to-eat cereals, fortified Salmon, cooked, 3 oz. (85 g) Sardines, canned in oil, drained, 1 oz. (30g) Tuna fish, canned in oil, 3 oz. (85 g)
Vitamin E	Corn Green, leafy vegetables Nuts	Olives Vegetable oils Wheat germ

Vitamin D

Recent discoveries indicate that vitamin D may be protective against some cancers with higher levels in blood associated with lower cancer risk in humans. This is best documented for colon and colorectal cancers where vitamin D emerged as a protective factor in a study of over 3,000 adults who underwent a colonoscopy between 1994 and 1997 to look for polyps or lesions in the colon. Vitamin D is also very important for calcium absorption and bone health. However, the National Health and Nutrition Examination Survey III surveyed vitamin D intake and blood levels of Americans and found significant deficiencies in many Americans. Low blood levels of vitamin D were found in 42.4 percent of African American women and 4.2 percent of white women.

Wrinkles

You may wonder if food can help your skin look less wrinkled. That very topic was the subject of the 2001 scientific article, "Skin Wrinkling: Can Food Make a Difference?" Researchers looked at the Swedish population aged 70 or older, and discovered that those who had a higher intake of vegetables, olive oil, and mono-unsaturated fat and legumes had less skin wrinkling. Also, those who had a lower intake of milk and dairy products, butter, margarine, and sugar products had less skin wrinkling. Although preliminary, these are interesting results. A similar study was performed in the United States looking at dietary nutrient intake and skin-aging appearance among middle-aged American women. This study found that higher vitamin C intake lowered the likelihood of a wrinkled appearance and dry skin. Also, higher linoleic acid intake, as found in vegetables, fruits, nuts, grains, and seeds, resulted in less skin dryness and less thinning of the skin. A 0.5 oz. (17 g) increase in fat and a 1.7 oz. (50 g) increase in carbohydrate intake increased the likelihood of wrinkles and skin thinning independent of age, race, education, sunlight exposure, income, menopausal status, body mass index, supplement use, physical activity, and energy intake.

Food and skin problems

Good nutrition and certain foods can improve your skin. Are there certain foods and beverages that can also worsen skin disorders? The data that support a certain food group causing the worsening of a skin condition are sparse; however, there are some skin disorders that seem to worsen if certain foods are consumed.

Acne vulgaris

Almost every day, patients will ask if there is something in their diet that is causing them to break out. They also ask if their diet is deficient in a nutrient or vitamin that may be responsible for their breakouts. For acne vulgaris, there are numerous studies that have proven no link between diet and the worsening of acne vulgaris. Recently, however, a study compared young men aged 15 to 25 who consumed a low-glycemic diet consisting of whole-grain cereals, barley, oats, and most fruits to a control group who had a diet rich in carbohydrates. After 12 weeks the men who had consumed a low-glycemic diet had a decrease in their acne lesions, as compared to the control group. In another study, more than 47,000 nurses with acne as teenagers were asked to complete a questionnaire about their diet while they were in high school. There was a positive association with their teen acne and a diet rich in milk (whole, low-fat, skim), instant breakfast drinks, sherbet, cottage cheese, and cream cheese. The study posits that the presence of hormones and bioactive molecules in milk contributed to the acne. It is important to note that more studies need to be carried out to confirm these findings before we recommend modifying your diet to improve your acne.

FOODS THAT MAY WORSEN ROSACEA SYMPTOMS
• Black pepper
• Garlic
• Hot sausage
• Hot peppers
• Paprika
• Red pepper
• Vinegar
• White pepper

Rosacea

There are some data implicating the role of certain foods in the worsening of rosacea. There are several important categories of dietary products that have the potential to cause this condition to flare. Rosacea is often triggered by hot beverages that range from tea to coffee to soups and ciders. Drinking lukewarm, as opposed to hot, beverages can help to minimize rosacea. Spicy foods such as Indian foods that are rich in curry, or foods with cayenne or hot peppers, are certain triggers. Certain types of alcohol, especially red wine, may also cause flares. Since there are other foods that can cause rosacea to flare, it is recommended that patients diagnosed with rosacea keep a journal to track their food and beverage triggers so they will know what to avoid. It is highly recommended that individuals with rosacea avoid the foods and beverages listed in the box above.

In general, botanical agents that have anti-inflammatory properties are good to use on inflamed, irritated, red, or itchy skin.

Eczema

There are also data that support the role of foods in flares of eczema. Foods reported to worsen eczema symptoms, in some people, include eggs, milk, peanuts, soy, wheat, and fish. Since each individual is different, there may be other foods that can cause your particular eczema to flare. To better understand and identify which foods may be triggers for you, it is important to keep a food journal. When your eczema begins to flare, write down all of the foods that you have eaten in the previous few days. Continue the list until after the flare has resolved. Then you can review the journal and identify possible triggers. If you still are unsure about your food triggers, an allergist can perform tests and even instruct you to eliminate certain foods from your diet and then re-introduce them to see if they trigger a flare.

Psoriasis

Psoriasis is known to flare after the consumption of alcohol. Also, alcohol may inhibit the effectiveness of psoriasis treatment. Therefore, moderate drinking for psoriasis patients is recommended, and if they suspect it is worsening their symptoms, they should avoid alcohol completely. A study performed in Italy reported that psoriasis improved with eating the following foods: carrots, tomatoes, and fresh fruits.

If you wish to alter your diet to improve a skin condition, it is important that you discuss the evidence supporting an improvement with your doctor. Do not listen to your best friend or the neighbor next door. You should avoid any radical diets that claim to cure your disorder.

Natural ingredients and home remedies

In today's world, despite scientific advances in treatments for skin problems, many people prefer to rely on both natural ingredients and home remedies. These remedies are preferred because they are readily available, easy to use, are gentle on the skin, and avoid the use of harsh chemicals. Most natural ingredients are botanicals, derived from plants. In many cases, conclusive

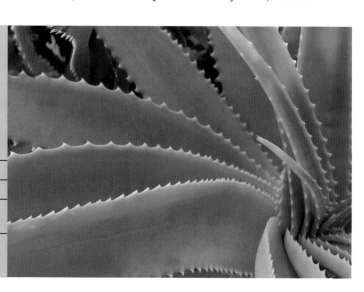

SKIN DISORDERS REPORTED TO IMPROVE WITH ALOE VERA

You may use the aloe plant directly from the garden. Simply snap or open the leaves and apply the gel directly on the skin.

- Eczema
- Psoriasis
- Dry skin
- Itchy skin conditions, like poison ivy
- Minor burns

scientific evidence of their effectiveness does not exist. However, many of these remedies have survived the test of time as they have been passed down from one generation to the next.

Aloe vera

Aloe vera is a plant that grows across the globe and is used in a variety of cosmetic and hair products. It has also been used extensively to treat a range of skin problems. The aloe vera plant is rich in mucopolysaccharides, amino acids, enzymes, and various minerals. Aloe vera has been shown to reduce inflammation in the skin, so it is widely used in much the same way as cortisone-containing creams, which also reduce inflammation. The ability of aloe to reduce inflammation is the reason that it is used to soothe conditions in which inflammation, redness, and itching are a key component. So the aloe plant is used for conditions, such as eczema and psoriasis, as well as superficial burns and poison ivy. Aloe vera has also been found to possess antibiotic and antiviral properties, which explains its use for treating minor skin infections. It is because of these properties that aloe is a popular ingredient in soaps, lotions, sunscreens, shampoos, and conditioners.

SKIN SOLUTION
Cocoa butter has been used by women for centuries to moisturize and soften their skin. Although conclusive proof does not exist, it has also been used as a home remedy for stretch marks and skin discolorations.

Baking soda

Baking soda, which is the alkaline chemical sodium bicarbonate, is a more natural and gentle ingredient used to treat several types of odor. You may be familiar with using baking soda in your refrigerator to absorb unpleasant food odors. Baking soda has also been used as an underarm deodorant, a foot deodorant sprinkled into shoes, and as a mouthwash. It can remove strong odors such as onions and garlic from hands. When mixed with hydrogen peroxide, it has been used as a toothpaste. When rubbed on elbows and knees, it can produce soft, smooth skin. Finally, baking soda may be used to soothe irritated and eczema-prone skin as well as to calm superficial burns.

Cocoa butter

Cocoa butter is actually a fat that is derived from the beans of the cocoa plant. It is best known as the ingredient that gives chocolate its flavor. Cocoa butter has been widely used in a variety of skin care products, but it is primarily used as a moisturizing ingredient for dry skin and as a treatment for itchy skin conditions such as dermatitis and eczema. It is formulated in lotions, oils, and creams as a general moisturizer and to maintain soft and smooth skin. Cocoa butter is a frequently used home remedy for the treatment of stretch marks during pregnancy. For individuals with darker skin tones, it is often used to lighten dark marks and discolorations on the skin. Some people use cocoa butter to soothe their sunburned skin.

Green tea

Green tea has become known as a very potent antioxidant. Antioxidants have the potential of calming inflammation in the skin and protecting from sunburn and skin cancer. The protective effects of green tea have been achieved by drinking the tea as well as applying it topically to the skin.

Milk

Milk, which is rich in fat, protein, and lactic acid, has been used on the skin for its beautifying and anti-inflammatory properties. Milk baths or milk-containing cleansers have been used for gentle, soap-free skin cleansing. The alpha hydroxy acid component of milk has popularized milk baths as a quick and easy way to soften the skin and remove the dead layers of skin. Silky, smooth skin will be revealed with this easy beautification technique. Finally, milk compresses applied to itchy and irritated skin will relieve the itching quickly due to its anti-inflammatory properties.

The benefits of alpha hydroxy acids on the skin were identified hundreds of years ago when Cleopatra was reported to have taken sour milk baths to soften and clarify her skin.

Oatmeal

Oatmeal is derived from the *Avena sativa* plant, and its skin benefits have been known and utilized for hundreds of years. Oatmeal is a grain that is rich in proteins, sugars, lipids, and minerals. It is used as a soap-free cleanser and is particularly useful for skin that is sensitive, dry, inflamed, or irritated. In addition to the ability to absorb dirt and skin oil, oats can repair damaged skin. Therefore, oatmeal is used to soothe and protect skin affected by dermatitis or eczema. Oatmeal is found in various formulations, although soaps, lotions, creams, and powders (to be dissolved in bathwater) are the most popular.

The oil of the tea tree protects the plant from bacteria and fungus. When used on human skin, it can also have a protective effect.

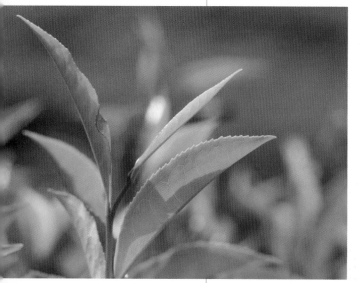

Olive oil

Olive oil is a relatively inexpensive and plentiful oil that is used as a moisturizer for the skin and as a conditioner for the hair. It has also been used for the treatment of dandruff in adults and for cradlecap in infants. Typically it is applied to the scalp and left on for about 15 minutes and then washed off, thus lifting the adherent flakes or scales.

Tea tree oil

Tea tree oil, derived from the leaves of the *Melaleuca alternifolia* plant, is useful for a variety of purposes. It has antibacterial, antifungal, antiviral, and anti-inflammatory properties. It has been used as a treatment for facial acne. In fact, one study has demonstrated that a tea tree oil gel is as effective as benzoyl peroxide 5 percent, although tea tree oil takes longer to work. Tea tree oil has also been used to treat several fungal infections including those of the feet, nails, and groin.

Vinegar

Vinegar is an ingredient that has also been used for the treatment of bacterial, fungal, and yeast infections. Its high acid content is responsible for these anti-infective properties. Vinegar has been used as eardrops for swimmers to prevent and to treat swimmer's ear. It does this by producing an acidic environment that retards bacterial overgrowth. Vinegar soaks can be used in the body folds and the nails and to prevent and decrease the growth of fungi and yeast. Vinegar soaks can also remove the green color sometimes present when fingernails and toenails have become infected with certain bacteria.

Vitamin E

Vitamin E, also known as tocopherol, is found naturally in vegetable oils, sunflower seeds, nuts, brown rice, and whole grains. Vitamin E is often applied directly to healing wounds to facilitate healing and to prevent and treat scars. It is also used to improve skin tone and texture. It is important to know that some people will develop an allergic reaction to topical Vitamin E applied directly to the skin.

Witch hazel

Witch hazel, derived from the shrub *Hamamelis virginiana*, has been used to treat itchy or inflamed skin. The shrub's bark and leaves have been used as a local anesthetic and astringent. It is commonly used as a cosmetic toner because the large quantities of tannins contained in witch hazel cause the skin to tighten, remove excess surface oil, and decrease bacteria particularly on acne-prone skin.

Yogurt

Plain yogurt, rich in protein, calcium, vitamins, and rich in alpha hydroxy

SKIN SOLUTION

A green discoloration of toenails or fingernails is often the result of an infection from the bacteria Pseudomonas. A solution of one part white vinegar and four parts warm water, used daily to soak the nail, will likely result in the fading of the green color.

Witch hazel applied to a cottonball is an inexpensive way to remove excessive debris and oil from the skin's surface.

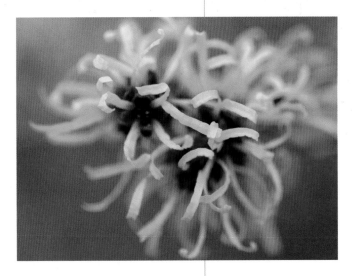

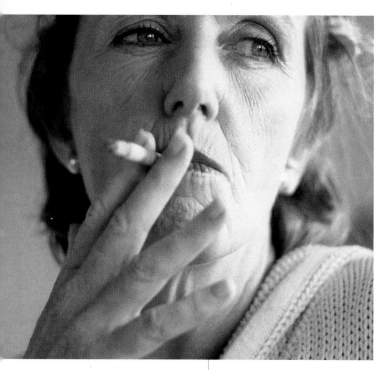

acids, makes it an ideal skin cleanser. It is also used as a facial mask to soften the skin.

Smoking and your skin

Smoking can affect your skin and how you look. Cigarette smoke produces free radicals that damage skin cells, leading to premature aging. It also reduces the supply of blood to the skin, and skin cells do not receive proper nutrients or enough oxygen. With premature aging caused by smoking, there is damage to the building blocks of the skin, collagen, and elastin. A reduction in both collagen and elastin leads to sagging of the skin and wrinkling.

Although wrinkles caused by smoking may appear anywhere on the body of smokers, wrinkles are most pronounced on the face and around the lips. A study that examined the facial skin and appearance of identical twins demonstrated that the twin who smoked had more wrinkles than the identical twin who did not smoke. Additionally, smoking thins the skin. Another study involving identical twins demonstrated that the smoker's skin was 25 to 40 percent thinner than that of the nonsmoker.

Also the skin may take on an abnormal or unhealthy color due to smoking. It may become yellow, reddish, or dark gray in color. Your face may develop a gaunt appearance. Fingertips and fingernails may become yellow or brown in color. It has been revealed that smoking one cigarette can reduce the flow of blood to the thumb by 24 percent. You may not realize that it can be unpleasant for a nonsmoker to be around smokers. The smell of the smoke lingers on your hair, breath, and clothing.

Smoking often accelerates the aging process, with prominent wrinkles around the mouth.

Smoking cigarettes, cigars, or pipes is harmful to the body and damages the appearance of your skin. Second-hand smoke can also lead to illness.

Exercise and your skin

Exercise can also have a significant effect on the skin. Just as with other organs of the body, exercise can increase circulation of blood and the delivery of oxygen and nutrients to the skin. This allows the skin to renew its building blocks of collagen and elastin. Often you can tell if people exercise regularly because they have better overall complexions and skin.

Acne

Exercise can improve a very common skin condition—acne. Acne is exacerbated by stress. Stress increases the production of several hormones in the body but particularly increases the male or androgen hormones, DHEA (dehydroepiandrosterone) and DHT (dihydrotestosterone). Increased levels of these hormones cause your skin cells to produce more oil or sebum, which then leads to increased growth of bacteria on the skin and plugging of skin's pores.

Exercise can have a positive effect on the skin, helping with acne, wrinkles, sagging, and color.

As you exercise, your stress level decreases and your body produces less of the androgen hormones that contribute to acne flare-ups. Some doctors think that as you sweat during exercise, you help to unclog your pores which, in turn, will help with your acne. Also, if you exercise, your acne will likely be in better control with fewer outbreaks and those that occur will be less severe and resolve quicker.

Antiaging

Exercise is also felt to have an antiaging effect on the skin. We know that as exercise increases the skin's supply of oxygen and nutrients, collagen and elastin are more readily produced. Renewed collagen will help with skin firmness and wrinkling. During and after exercise, your whole body relaxes, and your facial muscles do as well. This allows your crow's feet and frown lines to soften.

Exercise improves the color of the skin, giving a rosy glow as opposed to the yellow or gray color of those who do not exercise. Exercise may even help with cellulite on your thighs, buttocks, and legs. Stretching and toning muscles with weight lifting or with yoga or pilates workouts may reduce the appearance of cellulite.

Toxins

Exercise promotes good circulation that accelerates the removal of toxins from the skin and body. Everyday we are exposed to pollutants in the air from automobile exhausts, cigarette smoke, chemical plants, and refineries. These pollutants can be removed from the body and skin more quickly with exercise. Physical activity and exercise are recipes to achieving and maintaining good overall health and well-being. An added benefit is that it goes far in approving the appearance and health of your skin.

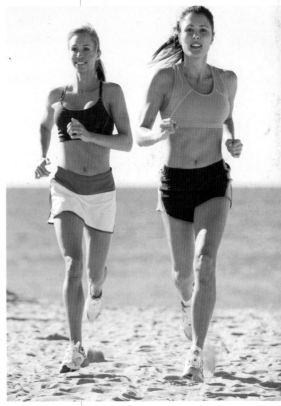

Daily exercise is important for skin health but don't forget to apply a waterproof sunscreen before engaging in outdoor physical activity.

Glossary

Abdominoplasty: surgical procedure to flatten the abdomen by removing extra fat and skin and tightening the abdominal wall muscles. Also known as a tummy tuck.

Acanthosis nigricans: velvety brown skin discoloration most commonly found on the neck of people who are overweight or who have diabetes.

Actinic keratosis: precancerous growth caused by sun damage characterized by a slightly rough patch of skin that may appear pink, red, or flesh-colored.

Anagen phase: active phase of hair growth cycle, generally continuing 2 to 8 years.

Androgenic alopecia: hereditary type of hair loss caused by hormones called androgens.

Angioedema: potentially life-threatening swelling of the tissues beneath the surface of the skin that often occurs on the face, mouth, or throat.

Antioxidants: substances that help stabilize or neutralize free radicals to prevent or reduce inflammation and subsequent damage to skin cells. See also free radicals.

Apocrine glands: sweat glands whose secretions are broken down by bacteria to cause body odor, primarily located under the arms and in the genital area.

Arbutin: widely used berry extract that is effective in lightening the skin.

Augmentation mammaplasty: surgical procedure to enlarge the breast by inserting implants under the breast tissue or muscle. Also known as breast enlargement surgery or breast augmentation surgery.

Basal cell carcinoma: the most common of all cancers, occurring mainly on sun-exposed areas of the skin; can appear as translucent, flesh colored, pink, or brown papules, sometimes with ulcerations.

Biopsy: test involving the examination of a small sample of skin under a microscope. See also punch biopsy, shave biopsy.

Blepharoplasty: surgical procedure to improve the appearance of the eyelid by removing excessive skin and fat pads and tightening the muscles.

Body dysmorphic disorder: mental illness causing a preoccupation with minor or nonexistent flaws in appearance.

Botox: see botulinum toxin.

Botulinum toxin: neurotoxin injected in very diluted concentrations into the muscles of the face to relax the muscles that cause wrinkles. Also known as Botox.

Breast augmentation surgery/ breast enlargement surgery: see augmentation mammaplasty.

Bromhidrosis: sweating that produces body odor.

Calcium hydroxylapatite: primary component of bone and teeth, used as the key ingredient in one dermal filler.

Catagen phase: rest phase of hair growth cycle, typically lasting a few weeks.

Cellulitis: skin infection involving the dermis and soft tissue, appearing with redness, swelling, warmth, and pain.

Chicken pox: see varicella.

Condyloma acuminata: sexually transmitted warts that occur in the genital or anal area. Also known as venereal warts.

Conjunctivitis: eye infection commonly called "pink eye."

Deep venous thrombosis: blood clot in the deep veins of the legs.

Dermal fillers: substances that are injected beneath the surface of the skin to reduce the appearance of wrinkles and to augment the volume of the lips and cheeks.

Dermatitis: a general term to describe a red, itchy rash resulting from inflammation of the skin. Eczema is a type of dermatitis.

Dermatologist: medical doctor who specializes in the diagnosis and management of skin, hair, and nail diseases.

Dermatophytes: fungi that infect the superficial layers of the skin anywhere on the body.

Dermatosis papulosa nigra: small brown growths appearing most often on the face and neck of darker-skinned individuals.

Dermis: layer of skin beneath the epidermis.

Dermoscopy: a method used to magnify and examine skin lesions.

DHA: see dihydroxyacetone.

Diabetic dermopathy: raised brown patches on the shins, usually the size of a pack of cards, that may signal diabetes mellitus.

Dihydroxyacetone: key ingredient in self-tanner. Also known as DHA.

Eccrine glands: sweat glands that help regulate body temperature, mainly located under the arms, on the palms of the hands, and the soles of the feet.

Eczema: see dermatitis.

Eflornithine: a cream that slows the growth of unwanted facial hair.

Electrodessication and cautery: procedure used to treat basal cell carcinoma by scraping with a curette and burning with an electric needle.

Electrolysis: permanent hair removal in which an electric current destroys the hair follicle.

Emollient: a moisturizer that leaves the skin feeling soft and smooth.

Endocrine system: group of organs that produce and secrete hormones that enable the body to function properly.

Epidermis: outermost layer of the skin.

Epidermoid cyst: harmless, firm, round growth located below the surface of the skin anywhere on the body.

Epilator: device used to pull out hairs.

Estheticians: an individual trained in skin care who performs facials, chemical peels, microdermabrasion, and waxing and can recommend appropriate skin care products.

Facelift: see rhytidectomy.

Fibroblasts: cells responsible for producing collagen and elastin that provide support, strength, and elasticity to the skin.

Folliculitis: inflammation and infection of the hair follicles.

Free radicals: unstable molecules generated by ultraviolet light, smoking, pollution, and normal cellular functions that produce inflammation that damages skin cells and leads to skin cancers and premature aging.

Gastric bypass: surgical procedure to reduce caloric intake by rerouting the small intestine to a small portion of the stomach.

Glutathione: common ingredient in skin lightening products in some countries; its effectiveness has not been confirmed.

Granuloma annulare: rash composed of pink rings of individual tiny papules that commonly occurs on the hands and feet.

Herpes zoster: see zoster.

Hives: see urticaria.

HPV: see human papillomaviruses.

Human papillomaviruses: group of contagious viruses that cause warts and other conditions. Also known as HPV.

Humectant: substance that attracts water and helps hydrate the skin.

Hyaluronic acid: a naturally occurring substance in the skin that is also a popular component of a dermal filler.

Hydroquinone: chemical that decreases skin pigmentation.

Hyperhidrosis: excessive perspiration.

Hyperpigmentation: dark areas on the skin caused by excessive melanin production.

Hyperthyroidism: condition caused by a hyperactive thyroid gland that may result in warm, moist skin and hair loss.

Hypetrichosis: excessive hair growth.

Hyponychium: area underneath the tip of the nail.

Hypothyroidism: condition resulting from an underactive thyroid gland, which can cause hair loss on the scalp and eyebrows, and dry skin.

Impetigo: common bacterial skin infection characterized by a yellow crust.

Iontophoresis: treatment for hyperhidrosis involving the administration of an electric current.

Intertrigo: inflammation involving the skin folds.

Keloid: exuberant growth of scar tissue beyond the boundaries of the original injury to the skin.

Keratinocytes: skin cells that make keratins, the proteins that give strength to hair, skin, and nails.

Keratosis pilaris: common condition characterized by small rough bumps on the upper arms and thighs resulting from a keratin plug in the hair follicle.

Langerhan's cells: cells that populate the epidermis and serve to activate the body's immune system to fight off microorganisms that penetrate the skin.

Laparoscopic adjustable gastric band: new procedure that places a silicone band around the upper part of the stomach to reduce its size. Also known as Lap-Band.

Lap-Band: see laparoscopic adjustable gastric band.

Lateral nail fold: protective area on the side of the nail from which a "hang nail" can form.

Lichen planus: common rash of small, purple papules that can affect the skin, mouth, genitals, nails, or scalp.

Linea nigra: dark line stretching from below the sternal bone to the pubic bone, common during pregnancy.

Liposuction: procedure that uses various techniques to remove fat cells beneath the surface of the skin.

Longitudinal melanonychia: dark line running the length of the nail. Also called pigmented nail band or pigmented nail streak.

Lupus: chronic autoimmune disease involving swelling, inflammation, and tissue destruction.

Mask of pregnancy: see melasma.

Mastopexy: surgical procedure to lift and reshape drooping breasts.

Melanin: pigment that gives skin, hair, and eyes their color and provides sun protection for the skin.

Melanocytes: skin cells located in the basal layer of the epidermis that produce melanin.

Melanocytic nevus: growth that appears on the forehead, cheeks, nose, or chin. Also known as a mole.

Melanoidin: brown pigmentation produced by self-tanners that is different from the skin's natural melanin.

Melanoma: a form of skin cancer that is often dark brown or black in color, asymmetric and irregularly shaped, and responsible for the majority of skin cancer deaths.

Melanosomes: packages of melanin found in the skin and nails.

Melasma: skin discoloration affecting the face, also referred to as the "mask of pregnancy."

Merkel cells: cells found mainly in the deepest layer of the epidermis that act as receptors for the body's sense of touch.

Microdermabrasion: form of superficial skin resurfacing involving the use of tiny crystals or a diamond wand.

Midline hypopigmentation: light spots that appear on the chest over the sternum.

Milia: tiny cysts that appear on the face.

Mole: see melanocytic nevus.

Molluscum contagiousum: common condition characterized by flesh-colored papules with a central indentation, caused by a pox virus.

Nail bed: soft, flat area at the base of the nail.

Nail plate: clear, hard keratin surface of the nail.

Noncomedogenic: does not cause comedones (acne).

Occlusive: ingredients found in moisturizers that coat the skin to prevent moisture loss.

Ochronosis: a side effect of long-term use of bleaching agents resulting in material deposited in the skin that makes it darker.

Otorhinolaringologist: medical doctor who specializes in conditions of the ear, nose, and throat.

Periorbital hypermelanosis: common condition that causes dark circles around the eyes. Also known as periorbital hyperpigmentation.

Periorbital hyperpigmentation: see periorbital hypermelanosis.

Phototherapy: treatment of certain skin disorders with ultraviolet light.

Pigmentary demarcation line: an abrupt transition from darker to lighter skin tone.

Pigmented nail band/streak: see longitudinal melanonychia.

Pityriasis rosea: common rash characterized by a round pink or salmon colored "herald" patch followed a few days or weeks later by oval spots over the skin.

Pityriasis versicolor: see tinea versicolor.

Polycystic ovarian disease: condition inhibiting normal ovary function and estrogen production that causes acne, facial hair, and thinning hair on the scalp.

Poly-L-lactic acid: volume enhancer used to improve facial wrinkles and sunken areas of the face.

Post-inflammatory hyperpigmentation: dark spots left behind after a skin inflammation, such as a resolving pimple.

Proximal nail fold: protective cuticle area at the base of the nail.

Pruritic urticarial papules and plaques of pregnancy: itchy rash in pregnant women characterized by pink bumps, hivelike spots, or small water blisters.

Psoriasis: disorder involving the skin and nails characterized by a raised pink or red rash covered by silvery scales.

Punch biopsy: type of biopsy that uses a small, round razor blade to obtain a cylindrical core of skin. See also biopsy.

Punctate keratoses: depressions that occur on the palms of the hand and soles of the feet.

Rhinoplasty: surgical procedure to reshape the nose.

Rhytidectomy: cosmetic procedure in which the skin is raised outward, the muscles are tightened, and fat and excessive skin are removed. Also called a facelift.

Rosacea: skin disorder characterized by facial redness, pink bumps, or dry eyes.

Scabies: highly contagious infection caused by the sarcoptes scabeii mite burrowing under the skin.

Sclerotherapy: injection-based procedure to treat varicose veins.

Sebaceous glands: glands that produce oil that act as the skin's natural moisturizer.

Sebaceous hyperplasia: enlarged oil glands.

Seborrheic keratoses: benign brown or tan growth with a surface resembling broccoli or cauliflower.

Shave biopsy: type of biopsy in which the doctor uses a scalpel or razor blade to plane off a small area of the skin. See also biopsy.

Shingles: see zoster.

Skin tags: harmless extra pieces of skin found on the neck, under the arms or breasts, or the groin.

SPF: see sun protection factor.

Squamous cell carcinoma: type of skin cancer characterized by pink patches or plaques that may be scaly; commonly occurs in sun-exposed areas but may also occur in scars, burns, and other sites of previous trauma.

Stretch marks: see striae distensae.

Striae distensae: lines on the skin that occur when the skin is overstretched due to pregnancy, rapid weight gain or loss, or bulging muscles. Also known as stretch marks.

Subcutaneous layer: fatty layer of skin below the dermis that helps insulate the body.

Sun protection factor: measure of ultraviolet B (UVB) protection in sunscreens and lotions. Also known as SPF.

Syndet: synthetic detergent.

Telogen phase: shedding phase of hair growth cycle, usually 2 to 4 months in duration.

Tinea versicolor: common, harmless rash caused by a superficial fungal infection, usually occurring on the chest, back, arms, and sometimes the faces, of young people. Also known as pityriasis versicolor.

Tummy tuck: see abdominoplasty.

Ultraviolet protection factor: measure of how well the clothing protects against ultraviolet A (UVA) and ultraviolet B (UVB). Also known as UPF.

UPF: see ultraviolet protection factor.

Urticaria: raised, pink, itchy areas on the skin. Also called hives.

Varicella: common rash consisting of small water blisters surrounded by red skin. Also known as chicken pox.

Vitiligo: condition in which the skin loses its pigmentation, causing white spots in small or large areas.

Wood's lamp examination: examination with a black light to evaluate pigmentation problems such as vitiligo.

Xantholasma: deposits of lipids that appear as yellow spots on or near the upper eyelid.

Zoster: painful, localized rash that is caused by the varicella virus, usually limited to one side of the body, and develops later in life. Also called herpes zoster and shingles.

Additional Resources

USA

American Academy of Dermatology

The American Academy of Dermatology seeks to promote and advance the science and art of medicine and surgery related to the skin while enhancing patient care.
www.aad.org
Phone:
(866) 503-SKIN (7546)
International:
(847) 240-1280

American Skin Association

The American Skin Association is a non-profit organization dedicated to raising awareness of the skin's vital role, advancing research, and educating and thus improving the nation's public health.
www.americanskin.org
info@americanskin.org
Phone: (212) 889-4858

The Coalition of Skin Diseases

The Coalition of Skin Diseases is a voluntary coalition of patient advocacy groups addressing the needs and concerns of people suffering from skin-related diseases. The coalition supports science and clinical research, generates awareness of skin disease, and supports the growth of member organizations.
www.coalitionofskindiseases.org
Phone: (202) 243-0115

The Foundation for Ichthyosis & Related Skin Types

F.I.R.S.T conducts research, raises funds for research, and provides information and emotional support for those affected by the disease.
www.scalyskin.org
info@scalyskin.org
Phone: 215-619-0670

The Inflammatory Skin Disease Institute

The ISDO provides patients, physicians, and caregivers with useful information about inflammatory skin disease. The institute conducts research, educates and provides support and advice on such topics as treatment options, treatment trends, and lifestyle issues.
www.isdionline.org
LaDonna.Williams@isdionline.org
Phone: (800) 484-6800, ext. 6321

The National Eczema Association

Supported by individual and corporate contributions, the National Eczema Association helps those suffering from eczema. The association provides information and education for both patients and medical professionals while conducting research and raising public awareness of eczema.
www.nationaleczema.org
info@nationaleczema.org
Phone: 415-499-3474

The National Rosacea Society

The National Rosacea Society is the world's largest organization dedicated to improving the lives of the estimated 14 million Americans suffering from this skin disease.
www.rosacea.org
rosaceas@aol.com
Phone: 1-888-NO-BLUSH

The Skin Cancer Foundation

The Skin Cancer Foundation is the leading skin cancer prevention organization. Their comprehensive website provides the most up-to-date skin cancer information and facts, detailing tips for self-examination and finding physicians in your area.
www.skincancer.org
Phone: (212) 725-5176

UK

The London Dermatology Centre

The London Dermatology Centre is run by leading dermatologists and plastic surgery consultants from major London teaching hospitals.
www.the-dermatology-centre.co.uk
Phone: +44 (020) 7580 7759
enquiries@the-dermatology-centre.co.uk

Harley Street Medical Skin Clinic

The clinic offers comprehensive, revolutionary skin treatments and procedures, using knowledge and best practice pioneered by leading specialists around the world.
www.harleystreetskin.co.uk
Phone: +44 (020) 7935 0986
enquiries@harleystreetskin.co.uk

British Association of Dermatologists

Established in 1920, the British Association of Dermatologists is a charity-run professional organization for Consultant, Trainee and Staff and Associate specialist dermatologists in the UK and Eire.
www.bad.org.uk
Phone: +44 (020) 7383 0266
admin@bad.org.uk

Screen4Life, Skin Cancer Screening

The clinic offers unique skin-imaging technology and a team of dedicated healthcare and logistics professionals.
www.screen4life.co.uk
Phone: (0)1474 702335
information@screen4life.co.uk

The British Skin Foundation

The British Skin Foundation is a registered charity dedicated to raising funds for skin disease research.
www.britishskinfoundation.org.uk
bsf@bad.org.uk
To make a donation email:
bsf@justgiving.com
Phone: 0845 021 2110

CANADA

Canadian Dermatology Association

The association is dedicated to the advancement of both aesthetic and medicinal surgery relating to the care of the skin, hair, and nails.
www.dermatology.ca

Canadian Skin Patient Alliance

The CSPA provides education, information, an online supportive community, and opportunities to create and join local support groups for all Canadian skin patients.
www.skinpatientalliance.ca
info@skinpatientalliance.ca
Phone: 613-422-4267

Environment Canada UV Index and Sun Protection

Information and educational activities relating to the effects of enhanced ultraviolet (UV) radiation on health and environment.
www.ec.gc.ca/regeng.htm
mailto:enviroinfo@ec.gc.ca
Phone: 1-800-668-6767 (in Canada only) or 819-997-2800

Health Canada Sun Safety Guide

Provides information on sunlight and UV exposure, plus educational materials on family sun safety.
www.hc-sc.gc.ca/hl-vs/sun-sol/index-eng.php

Canadian Cancer Society

The Canadian Cancer Society is an organization run by volunteers committed to both the eradication of cancer and the support and enhancement of the lives of those living with the disease.
www.cancer.ca
ccs@cancer.ca
Phone: (416) 961-7223

Eczema Society of Canada

Resources for persons suffering with eczema, including patient support, education, awareness, and research.
www.eczemahelp.ca
director@eczemahelp.ca
Phone: (905) 535-0776

Psoriasis Society of Canada

Up-to-date information on treatment, programs and services relating to psoriasis.
www.psoriasissociety.org
Phone: 1-800-656-4494

Rosacea Awareness Program

Support and information about rosacea, a skin condition that is estimated to affect two million Canadians.
www.rosaceainfo.com

INDIA

Sanche Clinic

The Sanche Clinic in Mumbai specializes in skin and laser treatment. Their focus is on scientifically treating the aesthetic functions of skin. The team of qualified cosmetic dermatologists provide skin counseling, analysis, and aesthetic enhancement.
www.sancheclinic.com
Phone: 26323434
Mumbai@sancheclinic.com

The Indian Association of Dermatologists, Venereologists and Leprologists

IADVL is one of the largest dermatologic associations in the world. The association is committed to the promotion and advancement of Dermatology, Venereology and Leprology.
www.iadvl.org
Phone: +91 571 2409940
secretary@iadvl.org

The Indian Society for Paediatric Dermatology

Formed in 1996, the Indian Society for Paediatric Dermatology (ISPD) aims to stimulate and promote medical and scientific research and to contribute to the education of trainees in dermatology and scientific workers in the field of paediatric dermatology.
www.ispd.in
Phone: 08457 2304000
drraghubir@yahoo.co.in

The Institute of Applied Dermatology

The institute of applied dermatology is a non-profit organization that treats filariasis through the effective combination of various systems of medicine.
www.indiandermatology.org
Phone: 04994-230116
iadorg@satyam.net.in

SINGAPORE

The Dermatological Society of Singapore

The objectives of the society are to advance the knowledge and practice of dermatology, to promote research, acquire and publish literature and scientific works in this area, and to promote regional and international co-operation in dermatology.
www.dermatology.org.sg
Phone: 65-9129 4583
info@dermatology.org.sg

The Specialist Skin Clinic

The Specialist Skin Clinic in Singapore is a specialist medical dermatologic clinic dedicated to the diagnosis and treatment of skin conditions.
www.specialistskin.com/sg
Phone: (65) 6734 1411
enquiry@specialistskin.com.sg

National Skin Centre

The National Skin Centre (NSC) is an outpatient specialist dermatological center with a team of dermatologists who can treat every skin condition. The NSC provides specialized dermatological services, trains medical students and post graduates, and undertakes research in dermatology.
www.nsc.gov.sg

MALAYSIA

The Dermatological Society of Malaysia

PDM is the official society for Malaysian dermatologists. The society aims to advance the knowledge of dermatology, promote research, and acquire and publish literature and scientific works.
www.dermatology.org.my
Fax: 03-7722 2617
info@dermatology.org.my

PHILIPPINES

The Philippine Dermatological Society

The Philippine Dermatological Society is dedicated to skin health.
www.pds.org.ph
Fax: 924-8877
eamcderma@yahoo.com

Index

Acknowledgments

Quantum would like to thank the following for the use of their pictures reproduced in this book:

Istock 5, 25, 34, 35, 37, 39, 41, 45, 55, 59, 61, 62, 67, 68, 69, 70, 73, 76, 84, 108, 115, 136, 154, 155, 155, 155, 157, 158, 160, 161

SPL 10, 12, 13, 16, 17, 18, 19, 21, 23, 24, 26, 27, 28, 30, 35, 37, 44, 48, 51, 56, 58, 74, 82, 82, 86, 87, 88, 89, 90, 92, 93, 94, 95, 96, 97, 98, 100, 101, 102, 105, 106, 107, 111, 112, 116, 120, 125, 126, 128, 131, 132, 134, 134, 135, 137, 139, 139, 140, 144, 145, 151, 153

Corbis 2, 11, 29, 32, 33, 36, 39, 43, 66, 78, 98, 109, 124, 127, 130, 143, 162, 163

Alamy 15, 20, 47, 49, 57, 59, 71, 75, 79, 91, 102, 104, 113, 121, 138, 141, 147, 149, 150

Mediscan 22, 52, 53, 103

Shutterstock 98, 99, 123